D1522459

THE

WILDERNESS

CURE.

BY

MARC COOK,

AUTHOR OF "CAMP LOU."

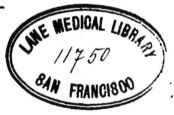

NEW YORK:

WILLIAM WOOD & COMPANY,

1881.

LAME LIBRARY

TROW'S
PRINTING AND BOOKBINDING COMPANY,
201-213 *East 12th Street*,
NEW YORK.

To

DR. WILLIAM H. WATSON

(Surgeon-General, and Regent of the University of the State of New York),

WITHOUT WHOM

THE WRITER WOULD NOT NOW BE,

NOR THIS LITTLE VOLUME EVER HAVE BEEN,

These Pages are Gratefully Inscribed.

NOTE.

THE publication of the article "Camp Lou," in *Harper's Magazine* for May, 1881, has called forth such a flood of inquiries that the author finds it quite beyond his powers to make individual reply to each. Precisely those minor details which could not well be embodied in a magazine paper have been most sought after by correspondents. This little volume, it is believed, contains the information desired. And it is given to the public in the hope that it will be accepted as a general response to the numerous letters which the writer has received on the subject of the Wilderness Cure.

CONTENTS.

THE WILDERNESS CURE.

CHAPTER I.

THE YOUNG MAN'S CASE.

LATE in the autumn of 1877, a young man at work in a newspaper office in New York City found himself the possessor of an inconsequential cough. It came to him unsolicited, and, so far as he could discover, without sufficient—certainly without specific cause. Up to that time he had enjoyed fairly good health. He had stood the strain of a reporter's life and boarding-house fare, and while pretty steadily disregarding the precepts of the doctors, he was never obliged to call upon them for prescriptions. It was not until he had found more congenial employment in the office of a weekly journal—not until he had sown his few wild oats, married, and settled down to the cultivation of tame oats, that the medical men got their grip upon him.

The inconsequential cough was scarcely noticed at first. It caused its owner neither inconvenience nor

1*

anxiety. In the consciousness of never having inherited anything, there was the comforting conviction that he could not have inherited consumptive tendencies. From no branch or root or twig of his genealogic tree was it possible to draw the wasting sap of phthisis. Still the cough, coming thus with no claim to kinship, stuck closer than a brother. At the end of a month or so, a physician prescribed some simple remedies. They were taken with no apparent effect. Another month went by. The cough had grown a trifle tiresome, but was still regarded as a small matter by its involuntary owner. It continued to be the only perceptible symptom of anything wrong. The young man lost neither flesh nor strength—at least, not to an appreciable degree. He went to the office, performed his usual duties without special effort, and was able to eat and sleep regularly. But he kept on coughing.

By the time the third month had been rounded the cougher had consulted other physicians, had taken three or four bottles of cod-liver oil, a gallon or two of rye whiskey with rock candy, and an amazing amount of good advice. The doctors found nothing very serious, they said, in the case. Perhaps a predisposition to pulmonary weakness—that was all. Exposure to the weather should be avoided, and possibly the climate of Florida or Nassau might prove of benefit. But there was no immediate necessity for leaving the city, and nourishing food, rest, and regularity of life would be pretty sure to overcome the trouble. So, still coughing, yet still free from anxiety regarding himself, the young man continued at his desk.

In March, 1878, some unpleasant accompaniments to the cough began to show themselves. Work became more exhausting, and a walk of a mile produced a strong desire for rest. The young man gave up the habit of mounting stairs two steps at a time. Tenderloin steak lost its old-time flavor, and indeed all eating became somewhat of a task. The pulse often rose to the nineties, and at times a slight fever manifested itself. Night-sweats were also developed, although in a mild form. All this time cod-liver oil, whiskey, and a diet of special nutritive qualities were continued perseveringly. And so was the cough.

On the first of April came the sharp warning which less alarming symptoms had failed to convey. On the evening of that day, after an especially laborious siege of it in the office, the cougher was attacked with hemorrhage of the lungs just as he stepped from the Fulton ferry-house. He raised, perhaps, half a teacup of blood. He had an idea, at the time, that it was a quart. This hemorrhage brought relief so far as the cough was concerned, but it brought also a tardy realization of the danger that threatened. The flow of blood was stopped by the use of common table-salt, and although the first attack was followed by a number of others, more or less severe, no other remedy was used. A day or two later, the young man locked his office desk and set forth in search of that unpurchasable luxury—

health. He went first to his father's home in the
central part of New York State. There he remained about two months, and then, in conformity
with the advice of his physician, Dr. William H.
Watson, the present Surgeon-General of New York
State, he journeyed to the White Mountains, New
Hampshire. The period between his departure from
New York and this mountain trip was marked by
some noteworthy peculiarities of his case. At first,
after his arrival at his father's house, he lost ground
at a discouraging rate. It was fully two weeks before the hemorrhages were completely stopped.
Meantime, his strength failed rapidly, the cough became extremely vicious, and the nights were made miserable through copious sweats, burning fever, and inability to sleep. In good time, however, matters began
to mend. Under the treatment of his physician the
patient regained his appetite, found the cough grow-
ing by degrees less troublesome, was able to sleep
restfully at night, and was entirely relieved from that
sense of nervous prostration which is not uncommon
in cases of hemorrhage.

So rapid was his gain, that in June the young man
had reason to believe that he should speedily be rid
of the cough which now again was the only reminder
of disease. On his way to the mountains he spent
a few days in Boston, and there submitted himself
to a thorough examination at the hands of Dr. G.
Hermann Merkel. The result of this examination
showed that the lower part of the left lung was
slightly consolidated, while the upper part of the

right lung gave some faint indication of catarrhal difficulty. Neither lung was in anything like a seriously diseased condition. Indeed, a less practised ear than the doctor's might have failed to detect anything wrong in the delicate tissues. Journeying on to North Conway, the health-seeker spent the remainder of the summer, where, from his window, he could see the giant front of Mount Washington. In the dry, bracing atmosphere of that region, where the sandy soil sucks up the moisture, and no foul odors pollute the air, he gained steadily. It was not easy, either for himself or others, to regard him as an invalid in those days. He led no life of piazza indolence. He turned off his allotted portion of work every day, and wrote with unusual ease and freedom. A three-mile jaunt did not tire him. Refreshing nights of sleep, and a regular appetite brought increased strength and added materially to his weight. And yet, through this cheering period, never, for a day, did the cough loosen its hold. At times, to be sure, it grew mild, and gave its victim long hours of respite; but all the same it was there. There to irritate, to watch its chance, and in the end to break forth again with renewed viciousness. In September the young man believed himself so far restored to health as to justify his return to New York. He turned the scales then at 158 pounds, a gain of twenty pounds over his weight in April. He felt in all respects as well, physically and mentally, as ever. His capacity for work and beefsteak was at its maximum. The physicians interposed no objections to his

return to office work. So he made his way back to
New York in the cheering belief that he had done
with cod-liver oil, quinine, and doctors' prescriptions.
But he took with him the cough.

In the next three months he attended regularly to
his duties, and did his best to shut out the too palpable truth that he was losing ground daily. At last,
however, the sharp warning was a second time
sounded. On the first of January, 1879, he was
taken down with severe hemorrhages. For the two
weeks following he was forced to keep his bed. All
the bad symptoms came back—nervous prostration,
weakness, loss of appetite, fever, debilitating sweats.
It was with the dawn of the new year that Dr. Edward W. Vietor, of Brooklyn, took charge of the
case. He gave the patient large hope of recovery,
and devoted himself faithfully to the work of bat-
tling the insidious enemy. It will ever remain the
conviction of the patient that without Dr. Vietor's
skilful treatment and the untiring care of a devoted
wife, his life would have ended at that time. As it
was, hope's thermometer rose and fell alternately for
many days. February found the young man seemingly on the straight road to recovery. And, indeed,
for a period of two months or more, he was well
enough to work daily, although not going to the office
—well enough to enjoy his meals, to find comfort in
books' companionship, and, in fair weather, in leisure-
ly strolls about town. But through some slight over-
exertion, added, perhaps, to indiscreet exposure, this
cheering condition of things was brought to a sudden

end. Toward the latter part of March a congestive chill was followed by something unpleasantly like pneumonia. Then for a month the patient ran down at an alarming rate. His physician saw the old foe gaining inch by inch, and foot by foot, until he felt the necessity for an immediate change of ground. The first thing was to get away from New York; the second was to get into the Adirondack wilderness. So weak, that he could with difficulty make the journey, the patient set out once more in the search for health—this time with very small hopes of finding what he sought. He spent a month at his father's home, hoping thereby to pick up a little strength for what, in his condition, seemed a laborious undertaking. Instead, however, of gaining, he grew steadily weaker. Dr. Watson, who renewed his interest in the case, joined heartily in the project of visiting the Adirondacks. He very plainly told the friends of the young man that this was the one chance left— that if it failed the long fight would be over. Enthusiastic as the doctor was over the Adirondack trip, he could not conscientiously hold out much hope in the present case. He made the fact emphatic, however, that the patient would die, and die speedily, if he remained where he was. Should he live to reach the St. Regis country, there was a chance—shadowy, no doubt, but still a chance—of recovery. Had the question been left for the young man himself to decide, the experiment would probably have remained untried. For it is to be confessed, that at this time (the early part of June, 1879), he had loosened his hold on hope and prepared himself, with what of philosophic calmness he could muster, for the coming of the end. Through many weary months he had held steadfast to the belief that he should find ulti- mate relief from his ailment; but now that belief gave place to one equally deep-seated, that death would claim its own. Cheering words from those nearest and dearest to him, even the blessed false- hoods which it is the physician's duty as well as privi- lege sometimes to utter, neither comforted nor de- ceived him. He needed no physician to tell him that he was sinking rapidly. And surely, with days made weary by the racking cough, with no appetite for food, with alternate fits of burning fever and chilling cold, with utter prostration of the nerve-force, with nights devoid of rest, the body drenched in perspira- tion, and the cough still racking the tired lungs— with all these things, it is not to be wondered at that hope went out, and the fight seemed altogether an uneven and vain contest.

Still the wiser opinion of others prevailed, and on the sixth of June the patient started for the wilder- ness. Plattsburg was reached that evening, and the night spent at a hotel. At an early hour the next morning the journey was resumed—twenty miles of it over a backwoods railway, and forty by stage over a backwoods highway. Only by means of alcoholic stimulants, freely taken, could the patient have made this trip. As it was, when he stepped from the stage at "Paul" Smith's, his wasted body and bloodless face afforded reason enough for the sturdy guides to shake their heads ominously over this doubtful specimen of a " sportsman."

That was the seventh of June. This is the middle of December. And the young man? Well, he lays down his pen to-day to go out for a seven-miles ride over the glistening snow. . The thermometer is close to zero. The air is crisp and cold. It might freeze your dainty city ears, but it is nothing to the hardy backwoodsman. Nothing to the young man.

CHAPTER II.

THE WILDERNESS AND THE EXPERIMENT.

DISTASTEFUL as it is to parade one's bodily infirmities before the world, such a course seems to be the only one to follow in a narrative like this. Indeed, my little volume would surely fail of its purpose if it did not have a personal story to tell. If this story should seem largely egotistical that is to be counted the misfortune, not the vanity of the teller.

The description of my own case given in the preceding chapter, however untechnical, is at least un-exaggerated. As it stands, it applies specifically to one victim; but with little alteration, no doubt, it would cover thousands of other cases. It has not been my object to make my condition worse than it was, nor shall it be my aim to color too rosily the curative virtues of the wilderness. The young man who, in June, found it no easy task to walk the length of the hotel piazza, in December could turn off a mile over snow-covered roads without exhausting his strength. But he is still far from robust health. The experiment has proved successful beyond the most hopeful anticipation, but it is to be remembered that it is an experiment still under trial. The man who has been afflicted with disease of twenty years' standing, and given up by the doctors, and who, after using six bottles of Dr. Lumbo's Liniment is, forthwith, able to lift a seven-octave piano, is not the writer of this book.   Probably all of us who are doomed to long familiarity with pills and powders, have, in one shape or another, been informed of the merits of innumerable Dr. Lumbos, each with his infallible liniment.   I regret to say, however, that personally I have never found that distinguished gentleman in the flesh, nor a drop of his liniment in the bottle.   I did not find them when I came up here into the woods.   Yet I heard of them—of a dozen of them—before I had got fairly settled in my room.

"D'yer want to know what 'll cure that there cough of your'n?" inquired a solicitous backwoodsman, before I had been three hours in the wilderness.

"Yes, it would afford me infinite satisfaction to learn what would cure that cough."

"Cherry-bark and balsam," was the impressive answer.   "Nothin' like it in the world!   Why, land o' the livin' there was a young feller come up here three years ago—"

But I spare you the proof of cherry-bark and balsam's magic properties, as illustrated in the case of that "young feller."   His case is painfully familiar. Sometimes it is cherry-bark and balsam, sometimes it is buttermilk, sometimes it is dandelion tea—but whatever the remedy, the result is invariably the same.   If any of my consumptive readers are emulous of the fame of Dr. Lumbo's patients, they will not come to the Adirondacks. I am persuaded, however, that there are in this country to-day ten thousand persons who, fighting the weary fight for health, would find cause enough for thanksgiving if they could penetrate this vast wilderness and breathe in the life-giving air day and night the year round. If it brought them that measure of strength which it has brought the writer, surely they, like him, would deem it a duty to write a recommendation of the medicine as sincere, if not as remarkable, as any ever given to Doctor Lumbo's Liniment.

The two weeks and more which we spent at "Paul" Smith's before getting into camp were wretched in the extreme. Nothing could have been worse than the weather. It rained almost incessantly the greater part of the time, and when not raining, it might with perfect consistency have snowed. The thermometer, on two or three occasions, sank below forty, and throughout it showed no more disposition to rise than the guides did when once seated about the office fire. Even the few enthusiastic anglers who had come in for the June fishing needed the warm glow of ardent zeal to keep them at their honored pursuit. As for a weak and shivering invalid, he could only move listlessly about his room, or hug the fire tenaciously in the parlor. If anything, I found myself worse during this fortnight than I had been at any time before. The nights especially became periods of almost continuous suffering. So hard and constant was the cough, that sleep, except the restless and troubled dozing produced by opiates, was out of the question. The expectoration was copious, generally of a greenish tint, and so solid that it sank like a stone in water. Then the drenching sweats, alternated with burning fever and occasional chills, made up a list of more ills than any flesh should at one and the same time fall heir to. We found kind friends at the hotel, and the sympathetic interest manifested in my case by "Paul" Smith and his estimable wife surprised me more then than it does now, when I have come to know them better. Dr. Trudeau, whose own case is referred to elsewhere in this book, freely gave his professional services in my behalf, and I was fortunate, also, in coming under the care of the late Dr. Bronson, of New Haven. All that medical skill and constant care and tender nursing could do was done for me at that critical time. If it did not surprise others, it did me, that I pulled through.

It had been a part of the wilderness plan, and a very important part in our preliminary arrangements, to go into camp at the earliest moment practicable. For myself, I had a very confused idea of what "camping out" meant. The plan was vaguely suggestive of salt pork, rubber blankets, a bed of hemlock boughs, and much physical discomfort, which is perversely declared to be fun. However, the camp was indispensable to a fair trial of the Adirondack experiment, and so our preparations were made with as much haste as possible.

In the matter of selecting a camping ground we were peculiarly fortunate. The spot was a bluff on

Osgood Pond, rising thirty feet above the level of
the water, and stretching like a peninsula into the
pond. Pines, spruces, and the aspen poplar, known in
the vernacular of the region as the "popple," abound-
ed. The pond itself stretched about this neck of land
so as to form a little bay, toward which the land extended in a gentle declivity. We thus had a breeze
blowing across the water in front to the water in the
back—a very important consideration in keeping clear
of insect pests. The spot had never before been used
for camping purposes, and that also was to be counted
in its favor. For custom gives the first settler a sort
of right of claim on Adirondack ground.

Our preliminary preparations were not elaborate,
and were left necessarily for the most part to the
guides employed to build the camp. We moved into
our primitive quarters on the 21st of June. We
found awaiting us two bark buildings and a canvas
tent, built in a line along the bluff, and facing the
picturesque little lake which nestles among the pine-
covered hills. Osgood is the first of the ponds lying
north of the Lower St. Regis, and is reached by a
three-fourths of a mile carry. To get to our camp,
another three-fourths of a mile had to be travelled
by boat; or the entire distance could be covered by
land, reckoned at about a mile and a half to the
hotel. It cannot be said that Camp Lou, as we afterward called it, presented a very attractive appearance on that first Saturday afternoon. To be sure
the scene about us was beautiful in the extreme; but
scenery was something which could not inspire us

much just then.   As I have explained, our fortnight's sojourn at the hotel had not in any way benefited me.   When I reached the camp, the walk up the gradual slope from the boat-landing to the tent was enough to exhaust my strength.   Despite the physicians' assurances, I looked with suspicion on the canvas tent, and very seriously doubted whether it would afford protection against the rain and wind. Timely advice had prevented us from putting our faith in hemlock boughs, and we had a comfortable bed, with mattress, pillows, and the other appurtenances of civilized sleeping.   But we slept very little that first night.   The weather was warm and mugny, with an unmistakable hint of rain in the lowering sky.   After an unrelished supper, we sat down disconsolately in the bark cabin and reflected that if this was the invigorating manner of life destined to restore health and strength, it was at least a questionable kind of invigoration.   The one tallow candle burned dimly, and was finally extinguished altogether to keep away the midges—which, if you want to be understood here, you must call midgets.   Our guides made a sorry attempt at enlivening the occasion by some reminiscenses of their backwoods life.   Then, finally, clinging stubbornly to my own belief about the insecurity of the tent, and finding that a drizzling rain had already set in, I insisted upon having the bed made up in the cabin.   This suited the midges exactly, and in the brief intervals of the night when the cough did not keep me awake, the persistent little insects did.

We arose on the following morning to find the
sky a mass of leaden clouds, and a penetrating rain
still falling. With the conveniences at our disposal
we made a rough and ready toilet and ate with doubtful appetite the breakfast which the guides had provided. Then wrapping ourselves in rubber coats, we
sat down in the tent, more discouraged and more
wretched even than on the night before. It was a
long, dull, miserable day, brightened only for an
hour by a visit from two of our hotel friends, whose
goodness of heart prompted them to brave the abom-
inable weather and seek us out to make sure that we
still lived. That night we took to the tent, our former experience having satisfied me that the bark
cabin was not a place for sleeping. And here came
the first convincing proof of the benefit I was to
derive from camp life. I found the tent as condu-
cive of sleep as the cabin had been antagonistic to
its enjoyment. To those accustomed all their lives
to the stifling atmosphere of the ordinary chamber,
it would be impossible to convey an adequate idea of
the delicious purity of the air as inhaled under canvas. Always as fresh as if out of doors, the tent
still shields the sleeper from the wind, and makes a
draught, that everlasting promoter of colds, an im-
possibility. From that first night I became an enthusiast over canvas coverings. Nor were my fore-
bodings with regard to the leaking of the tent in a
single instance verified. Throughout all the four
months and a half which we spent in camp, not once
did the rain penetrate the tent. And this was due to

no lack of test, for we had days when the drenching storms were enough to put the best shingled house to a severe trial. Moreover, our tent was neither new nor exceptionally secure. It was purchased at second-hand of a guide, and had done service for two or three years. The "fly" which protected it was made of ordinary cotton cloth and afterward immersed in linseed-oil.

For the first four weeks of camp life the only perceptible improvement in my condition was in the matter of sleep. Although still troubled at intervals by the cough, and by no means exempt from the sweats, still as a whole the nights brought a measure of rest which I had not known for many weeks. I had hoped to find a keener appetite for food in this out-door life, and some abatement of the cough. I cannot say that I expected these results, but the faith of others was so great that it gave me at least hope. But no such cheering symptoms manifested themselves. The cough—except, as I have already explained, during the night—remained as vicious as before. The fever became more constant, and that in the face of large doses of quinine recommended by the doctors. Instead of gaining, my appetite grew less and less, until most of the nourishment taken was in the form of beef-tea, milk, and raw eggs. Occasionally the sputa was colored with blood, and I was continually apprehensive of hemorrhage. Without energy enough even to find solace in reading, I passed the days listlessly in a chair, with no other desire than to be let alone.

2

So passed the first month. The weather was variable and very different from what I had been led to expect. The Fourth of July, for example, came and went, while we shivered over a roaring fire. Two weeks later, a hot wave struck us, which sent the mercury up among the nineties, even in the coolest spot of our pine-shaded ground. Along with these sudden and extreme changes of temperature, came a great deal of rain and some wind. The insects did what they could to bother us, and our lack of experience cost us many petty annoyances, which would seem silly to enumerate, but which are not trivial to the invalid.

With the second month a gain, very slight, but still appreciable, began to show itself. There were days when I could eat with fair relish, when the fever was wholly absent, and when my energy was sufficiently aroused to do a little work in the way of writing, and to take some slight physical exercise. Sometimes these good turns would cover a period of three or four days. Oftener, however, they gave way at the end of twenty-four hours to a condition wherein all the worst symptoms displayed themselves anew. At my best, it must be remembered that the cough was always present, and always persistent. At my worst there were also the fever, the nervous prostration, and a miserably impaired digestion.

At the close of the third month, that is, toward the latter part of September, I had made some unmistakable progress. With rare exceptions I sat down to my meals with a good appetite. I could walk half a mile without overtaxing my strength. Patience, atropine, and the pure air of the tent had about mastered the sweats. The nights, although sometimes wakeful, were still restful. I spent an hour or two every day in writing, and kept in motion enough to give me a fair amount of exercise.

From this time to the breaking up of our camp, November 3d, I continued to pick up a little, albeit a backward wave would at intervals strike me and temporarily chill my hopes. But when we took down the canvas tent in a driving snow-storm, nineteen weeks after we had first slept under its shelter, I felt that the camp life experiment had proved a success. I had gone in miserable, indifferent, and skeptical. I was not cured; but I came out comfortable, alive, and full of hope.

CHAPTER III.

SOME DELUSIONS DISPELLED.

WHEN we first came into the wilderness, or more strictly speaking, when the idea of coming was first decided upon, a little definite information would have been of much practical value. A knowledge of what was needed for the trip, of what ought to be done after we had reached our destination and of what manner of life it was that we were to lead, would have saved us an undetermined amount of annoyance, disappointment, and unnecessary expense. In short, if some other fellow had recorded his experience before the summer I went into the woods, I should have blessed him, and I should not have written this little book.

The physicians had said, "You must go to the Adirondacks and camp out." Very well. The Adirondacks it is. And a very little investigation was enough to show that the particular spot to go to must be "Paul" Smith's. So far the programme was simple. But at this point all exact information came to an abrupt end. There were the doctors themselves, but they had never visited "Paul" Smith's, and never camped out. Besides, they were not supposed

to be encyclopedias of backwoods lore. Their duty
ended with the command to go. There was Dr.
Loomis's paper in the *Medical Record*. This I got
hold of and read with profound interest, but while it
gave large cause for hope, it left all minor details
untouched, and confined its narrative to that simple,
technical style, characteristic of the medical professor.
There was the Rev. Mr. Murray's book. That certainly ought to contain some important facts. So I
secured a copy and read it diligently. Facts I found,
and some very excellent reading to boot; but the
possible tourist of Mr. Murray's imagination could
not be an invalid. He was to journey over long
" carries," run rapids, penetrate the unexplored forest, and shoot a deer whenever he was hungry. He
was to provide himself with a rifle, with strong
woollen trousers, a pair of woollen shirts, two pairs of
woollen socks, soft felt hat, top boots, a rubber overcoat, and plenty of woollen blankets. This super-
abundance of woollen seemed a little mysterious for
midsummer wear. But for Mr. Murray's traveller it
was undoubtedly the thing. Mr. Murray further in-
structed his reader to make a bag of muslin in which
to tie up his head and thus shield it against insects,
and to procure a pair of stout buckskin gloves with
gauntlets, along with a copious supply of tar and
sweet oil. To his lady tourist he recommended short
flannel skirts, Turkish trousers, and a soft hat like a
man's. All this was undeniably good advice, but it
did not exactly meet the case of the invalid.

From Mr. Murray we turned to a dozen other

books bearing upon the wilderness, but found only a
repetition of the woollen, gauze bags, and tar oil.
Nobody apparently had prepared for other than robust travellers in his calculations. It did not seem
safe to wholly ignore these numerous warnings, and so
we burdened ourselves with many useless things that
are never needed here nor elsewhere. I may be pardoned if I undertake to dispel a few of the popular
delusions which have long been cherished with respect to the Adirondacks, and which, when once removed, may make the tour for health appear more
inviting.

To begin with, "camping out" may be absolutely
dissociated from salt pork, the frying-pan, and all
other abominations. One may surround himself,
forty miles in the wilderness, with all the comforts,
and nearly all the luxuries, that he might enjoy in his
own city home. This assertion is made, of course,
on the assumption that the camp is to be permanent,
and pitched within easy access of some one of the hotels. In these pages all the facts given relate to the
St. Regis region, of which "Paul" Smith's may be
considered the centre. Perhaps other parts of the
wilderness afford equal advantages to the seeker after
health: but it will be my purpose to deal with those
matters only which come within range of my personal experience. A camp, then, situated within a
radius say of three miles from the hotel, can be made
thoroughly comfortable. And this is what is meant
by comfort:

A tent affording complete protection against rain

and wind. A good bed in which you may sleep between sheets, and in proper night-garments. Two or three bark buildings, one of which may be used as a sitting and lounging room, when the weather is unpropitious; another as a dining-room, and a third as a kitchen. A small storehouse for garden implements, tools, etc. An open arbor, at the water's edge an ice-house. In your tent and buildings well-laid floors, a stove to take the chill off, if the night grows cold, tables, chairs, books, writing utensils, a student lamp, a clock, and such other conveniences as you may desire. A good table, with a menu embracing anything you want, from bouillon to ice-cream. A daily mail. Wine and lager beer, stowed in the cool bank of sand. A boat to glide over the picturesque lake when you feel so disposed. The great forest about you, through which the wind comes laden with the rare odors of pine and balsam. A cigar in the evening as you sit in front of a blazing log fire, which roars and crackles and makes fantastic shadows among the giant trees. Freedom—delicious, absolute freedom—from dust and noise, and the roar of city streets.

There is an idea of comfort.

But there are other mistaken beliefs regarding the wilderness besides that which makes camp life a hardship. Those who have drawn their information from books, instead of experience, are pretty apt to pin their faith on one of two extremes. Either they picture the Adirondacks as a place where wild beasts still rove at large, or else they speak of it disdain-

fully as the resort of embryo sportsmen who never
shoot off their guns for fear of blackening the silver
mountings.   Both of these extremists should come
up into the woods and look about them with discern-
ing eyes.   They would concede, probably, that the
best hunting and fishing in New York State are to
be found here.   Whether what is best in New York
would be more than tolerable in the far West admits
of doubt.   The man who penetrates these woods for
the first time, expecting to find deer browsing in
herds, and schools of trout awaiting impatiently the
delusive fly, will be sadly disappointed.   There are
deer here, undoubtedly—deer to be shot, if the hunts-
man is possessed of patience and skill enough to
shoot them; but observation quickly convinces one
that these timid animals do not invite self-destruc-
tion by holding conventions in conspicuous places.
There are trout here, too, any number of them; but
they are wise in their generation, and will not, as a
rule, accept every fly that is cast with unquestioning
confidence.   From our own tent door we have seen
three tempting bucks at one time drinking in the
lake.   And yet it was generally difficult to get hold
of venison throughout the season.   An expert and
genial angler brought in, during our sojourn at the
hotel, a speckled trout which actually weighed five
pounds and a half.   The skeptical reader may satisfy
himself of the truth of this assertion, whenever he
enters " Paul" Smith's, for the rare fish is preserved
in a glass case in the office.   And yet, in spite of this
palpable proof of what the Adirondack waters con-

SOME DELUSIONS DISPELLED.   33

tain, other expert fishermen may cast the fly all day
and land nothing bigger than a nine-ouncer. Briefly
put, game and fish are here, but they are not to be
had for the asking.

So far as the insect pest is concerned, it would not
be right to count it among the delusions ; but, as has
already been intimated, it is by no means the evil
generally represented. If one is careful in the selection of a camping spot, making it a point to find high
ground, overlooking the water, he need not worry
much about the insects. It would be unjust to rob
the Adirondack bugs of any of the glory which right-
fully belongs to them, but, certainly, their achieve-
ments in the past have been grossly exaggerated. I
have known mosquitoes—known them intimately and
to my sorrow—which, dwelling in the modest retire-
ment of a Brooklyn boarding-house, could do more
effective work in five minutes than their Adirondack
fellows can in five weeks. The black flies which
come early in the season, and disappear almost wholly
by the first of July, were scarcely seen by us in camp.
Midges are certainly a nuisance, but a very slight
breeze is enough to carry them off, and this breeze
we generally enjoyed. It may be necessary, occasionally, to resort to the smudge—that is, a half-
smothered fire, kindled in an old pan or pail, and
placed in the tent long enough to smoke out the
winged nuisances—but, as a rule, the pollution of the
atmosphere caused by this remedy is more to be
dreaded than the evil itself. A mosquito netting to
cover the bed should always be provided. Yet even
2*

this will be found unnecessary after the first week of
September, and from that time forth no trouble need
be apprehended from any sort of insect.

A few years ago it was a common thing to run
across a bear anywhere in the St. Regis region. So,
at least, the veteran guides declare, and doubtless
there is some foundation for the assertion. But all
the accounts of wild beasts in the woods to-day are
to be accepted with caution, if accepted at all. The
tourist might travel through the very heart of the
wilderness, and, indeed, spend his life in so travelling, without once setting eyes on any animal more
ferocious than the deer. The wild beast feature may,
therefore, be entirely eliminated from Adirondack
life.

Then, again, although a camp should be pitched
forty miles in the wilderness, the dweller therein
would not be shut out from communication with the
world. He will get his mail regularly every day
through the hotel, and he will find the telegraph
wires at his disposal. He may read Monday morning's papers in his tent Tuesday afternoon. If urgent
reasons should make it necessary for him to return
at once to civilization, he can take his departure at
eight o'clock in the morning and awake the next
morning in New York. This consciousness of proximity to the outer world, while one is seemingly shut
up in the primeval forest, does much to reconcile the
invalid to his new life. He is comforted, too, by the
reflection that skilful medical aid, if such should be
needed, is within reach; for, apart from Dr. Trudeau,

whom the year-round inhabitants are proud to regard as belonging to the country, there is scarcely a week during the camping-out season, when one or more physicians may not be found at the hotel. Dr. Loomis owns a cottage within a stone's throw of the St. Regis Lake House, in which he spends a month or two every summer. The consumptive does not come into the wilderness to dose himself with medicine, but it is nevertheless a good thing to have a trustworthy physician within easy call.

Adopting the theory which is held to by most of the medical authorities of the day, that phthisis is a disease which calls for an abundance of the most nutritious food, the invalid in the woods finds himself in a peculiarly fortunate position. For here he may obtain, with comparatively little trouble, almost anything he desires to eat. Through the supply-store in the hotel, the delicacies and dainties of the table are at his disposal. Beef, mutton, and poultry are always to be had. In its season, venison, while not superabundant, can generally be obtained as often as the patient craves it. Speckled trout, fresh from the clear waters of the mountain streams, are as plentiful as smelts in Fulton Market. Later, the partridge tempts the appetite, and is supplied at surprisingly cheap rates. Fresh eggs, pure milk, and excellent butter are all to be had from the inhabitants or hotel. In short, if good living ever enables a man to conquer consumption, this is the place to find it.

Briefly, then, to recapitulate: this wilderness experiment need entail no hardship, no privation, and, as I shall show hereafter, only a very moderate outlay of money. In setting out on the journey the invalid need not encumber himself with any of the extraordinary equipments enumerated in the guidebooks. He may rest assured that his camp-life can be made comfortable and even luxurious. He has the word of the writer, given after full and fair experience, that a bed in a canvas tent is one of the delicious things in this life which, after trial, can never be forgotten. If his strength permits, and his taste runs in that direction, he may be sure that he will find fair hunting and excellent fishing in the St. Regis region. On the contrary, if he is too much of an invalid to indulge in these pursuits, or if he has no fondness for them, he may solace himself with the reflection that others will gladly provide him with fish and game. If a lady, nervous and timid, she may put the wild beast bugbear out of mind once and for all. As for the flies and mosquitoes, they are too trivial an annoyance to be seriously considered. The patient is not shut off from communication with the outer world nor from agreeable companionship. He is not put beyond the reach of skilful medical attendance. He is not obliged to forego the pleasures of the table. In a word, he is not compelled to make any great sacrifice in return for the precious privilege of breathing in, by night and by day, this God-given, life-saving air.

CHAPTER IV.

PREPARATIONS FOR AN INVALID'S CAMP.

LET it be supposed that the searcher after health has made up his mind to give the Adirondack experiment a trial. This conclusion should be reached, of course, only after consultation with a reputable physician. For it is always to be borne in mind, that while the more apparent symptoms of what is called consumption bear a close resemblance in pretty much all cases, yet the treatment required for one may be very different from another. And certainly it is not the purpose of the writer to persuade others to try the experiment of the woods unless with the consent of a doctor in whom the patient himself has confidence, and under whose advice he acts.

Supposing, however, the advice to have been given, and the trip determined upon. For its preparation, as has been already said, no extraordinary steps need be taken. If a man, the invalid will pack his trunk with such articles as naturally suggest themselves for a sojourn abroad of six months or a year. The only deviation from the usual necessities should be made by substituting woollen shirts for those which need the laundryman's skill before wearing. Linen cuffs

and collars may be dispensed with, and a plentiful
supply of underclothing and woollen socks provided.
It is a good thing, too, to have a night-dress of flannel, long and loose. In the case of a woman, it would
be presumptuous to dictate her wardrobe, but she
may safely leave behind her the Turkish trousers
and gauze bags. For anybody, the simple direction
to take plenty of good warm apparel is enough.

From whatever point the tourist sets out, unless it
be from Montreal or that part of New England which
lies nearer to Lake Champlain than to Boston or
Albany, he should make Saratoga his objective point.
Thence the journey to Plattsburg may be accomplished all the way by rail, in something less than
six hours; or a steamer may be taken at Whitehall
by those who care to get a better view of the picturesque Lake Champlain. Plattsburg is well provided
with hotels, and a pleasant rest of a day or two may
be taken there, if desired. The distance to St. Regis
Lake is about sixty miles. At present, twenty of
this is made by rail, and the remainder by stage. It
is expected, however, that before the close of the
summer of 1881 this stage ride of forty miles will
be shortened by more than one third—the railroad,
which was built by the State to the Clinton Prison,
having been extended so as to bring it to a point
twenty-four miles from " Paul " Smith's. It remains
now only to cut a carriage-road through the woods
from the terminus of the railroad to the hotel.
However, the invalid need not be frightened out of
coming at the prospect of travelling over the old route.

He will find the stage ride much less irksome than
he supposes, and if too weak to make the entire trip
in one day, he may stop over at the half-way house,
which is reached about noon, and which supplies the
traveller with dinner. If the invalid chooses to push
ahead, he will be set down at " Paul " Smith's somewhere about five o'clock in the afternoon.

It is safe to assume that pretty nearly everybody
who has heard of the Adirondacks has heard also
of Paul Smith's. Indeed, the definiteness with which
that name is fixed in the tourist's mind causes him
to stare with rather a nonplussed expression at the
sign which greets his eyes when he first steps from
the stage on to the piazza of this remarkable hostelry.
Can it be that he has gone astray and brought up at
the wrong spot? If not, why is the sign over the
door " A. A. Smith," instead of " Paul " Smith ?
When he comes to solve this riddle, he learns that
the genial backwoods landlord was originally named
Apollos Austin. The Austin was condensed to an
A., and the Apollos abbreviated to Polly, which in
good time reduced itself to Pol. This stood the test
of some years, but finally, by precisely what system
remains unknown, evolved itself into Paul. To-day,
the owner of the double-vowel initials repudiates
them both and recognizes himself only as Paul. This
metamorphosis in name is less remarkable than that
in the landlord's surroundings. Twenty years ago,
when " Paul " Smith put up a frame building of
modest dimensions to accommodate the stray sportsmen who occasionally drifted through that part of the

wilderness, he would have counted twelve lodgers on a single night as indicative of amazing prosperity. Now, in what is called "the season," more than three hundred guests often find accommodation in the house. By successive stages of growth—periodic additions of wings and Ls—the original tavern has stretched itself into the proportions of a first class summer-resort hotel. Indeed, its wings are so absurdly out of proportion to its original body, that it presents a butterfly appearance to those who knew it of old. The general verdict of all who make the hotel their headquarters is that it sets an excellent table, and furnishes every comfort which in reason can be expected. The rooms are neat and attractively furnished, the beds what they should be, the attendance good, and the general atmosphere of the house pleasant and homelike. But above all this, to the person accustomed to a city hotel, the thing which makes the deepest impression—which leads him always to return to "Paul" Smith's, after he has been there once—is the unaffected kindness of the landlord and his wife. In this there is not the slightest flavor of obsequiousness, nor a hint of mercenary motive. In evolutionizing from Apollos to Paul, in the transition from buckskin to point-lace surroundings, the man himself has not changed. No one is ever more welcome than he when the big parlor is crowded with fashionably dressed women and velvet-coated sportsmen. Yet if you want to find "Paul," you must look elsewhere than here. The simplicity of his nature, which is in nowise allied to simpleness, would be refreshing in any man. It is absolutely irresistible in the proprietor of a " fashionable " hotel.

For, I grieve to say, that Paul Smith's has become an undeniably fashionable resort. You will find less vulgar display than at Saratoga, but you will also find more solid wealth and more genuine purse-aristocracy. Precisely why these robust ladies put themselves to the inconvenience of penetrating the wilderness for the purpose of displaying their diamonds on the hotel-piazza, of reading a novel or lounging lazily in their rooms, of playing a mild game of whist and eating three hearty meals a day, is a mystery. For, although fashionable, St. Regis Lake affords most limited opportunities for the display of wealth where it can be seen of others. The year-round inhabitant is certainly an unpromising subject to undertake to dazzle. The man who has never seen a train of cars in this age is not to be made envious by diamonds or the most elaborate of toilets.

The fashionable element, however, is not to be counted a drawback in the case of the invalid. On the contrary, it is much better that he should be set down on the gay piazza of the hotel, where laughter and bright faces and the hum of many voices tell of the pleasures of life, than that he should find his destination a sanitarium pervaded by the odor of the sick-room. The very presence of these thoughtless, sound-lunged persons often proves a kind of tonic. His cough brings no sympathetic response from any fellow-sufferer—only a kind of brazen stare from the man with the athletic chest and the friar's digestion; and that stare awakens the invalid's resentment, and causes him to struggle with the wretched indication of his ailment until he strangles it for the time being.

As to the length of time to be spent at the hotel before entering upon the experiment of camp-life, that must, of course, be largely determined by circumstances. If the patient's strength permits, there is no reason why he should not be established in his tent within a week after his arrival. But should his condition be more critical, it may be necessary to delay the removal to camp until the bracing air has done something toward building up the wasted powers. In rare instances, where the disease is far advanced, it may not be advisable to try the camp-life at all, but in lieu thereof, to remain permanently at the hotel. In any event, it will be best to leave the question of camping-out to the physician—not necessarily to the home doctor, but to some one of the faculty who is personally familiar with this manner of life. For our present purpose, let it be assumed that the invalid is strong enough to try the camp as soon after his arrival as the necessary preparations can be made. What steps shall he take to best accomplish his object ?

First.—It is all-important that the invalid should secure the services of a faithful, competent guide. That word is used in conformity with the vernacular of the wilderness. As a matter of fact, there is very little "guiding" required by the person who is hunting for health. But as all the men who offer their services are called guides, the word may be used to avoid confusion. A good guide, then, is the first essential thing to find. And this question, like many others, may be advantageously left to the managing clerk of the hotel, Mr. Charles E. Martin.

Second.—The selection of a guide once made, the next step will be the choice of a spot whereon to pitch the camp. In deciding this question it should be kept in mind that the point chosen ought not to be more than a mile or two from the hotel, that it should be on high ground, as nearly surrounded by water as possible, and as abundantly supplied with trees as may be. Plenty of such places may be found on the Upper and Lower St. Regis Lakes, on Spitfire and Osgood Ponds. It were much wiser to build a camp within five hundred feet of the hotel—and many of them might be built within such a radius—than to strike out too far from the centre of supplies. High ground is to be looked to, not so much to avoid dampness, for there is no dampness worth speaking of in the region, as to keep clear of insects. The proximity of pine and balsam trees is a most desirable thing, whether regarded from the medical point of view or as a matter of mere comfort. For it should not be forgotten that even in the Adirondacks there are days when the sun blisters the earth and makes shade most welcome. The camping-ground should invariably border the water, not only because of the invigorating breeze thus obtained, but also because the mountain lakes are the highways over which most of the travel is accomplished.

Third.—We have now the guide and the camping-ground. In the sequence of importance, the tent stands next. This is so prominent a feature of the whole experiment, that it will richly repay the invalid to provide himself with the best. If two persons are to occupy the tent, it should be not less than 12 feet square. 12 by 14 feet is perhaps a better size. If the camper-out is alone, the canvas will serve its purpose if it measures 8 by 10 feet. Yet, even for one person, the larger size is much to be preferred. In case there is no question about the invalid's ability to go into camp immediately upon his reaching the wilderness, then it would be an excellent plan to purchase a tent before setting out on his journey. Otherwise, he may either order one after his arrival, or, if his sojourn is uncertain, he may hire one from the hotel. Large or small, the tent should be of the shape known as a wall tent, sound and whole, and protected by a "fly." The interior should always be floored, and provided with a stove. For the rest of the furniture the taste of the occupant must decide. A serviceable bedstead can be constructed by the guide out of poles, but the tourist should see to it that he is provided with a good mattress or two, pillows, and plenty of warm bedding. In place of an under mattress, boughs of balsam or hemlock may be used, a covering of stout cloth being first stretched over the bedstead. If the guide possesses the usual ingenuity of his class, he will be able to build tables, chairs, a lounge, and many other useful articles of furniture.

Fourth.—Apart from the tent, the only building absolutely necessary to the carrying out of the camp-life experiment is a kitchen, which may be so divided as to afford accommodations for the storage of provisions. It is better, however, on some accounts to have a separate storehouse or pantry, as the guide calls it; but this is a matter of individual preference. Some sort of a place in which to cook, however, is indispensable. Such a place can be put up in a day by two competent men. If to be used only as a kitchen, a bark building, say six feet by eight, will serve all purposes. These bark buildings, which can be made to display no little architectural beauty, are constructed on a frame-work of poles and boards, to which latter the bark is nailed. It is best to floor the kitchen, and, indeed, all the buildings of a permanent camp, with boards; but, except in the case of a tent, it is not a necessity. A good cook-stove should be the first and chiefest adornment of the kitchen. They have some theories here, indigenous to the country, of cooking by an open fire out of doors. The idea is poetical, but the palpable results are smoky. Let the kitchen be furnished with all the utensils usually found in such quarters, and let the frying-pan be hung so high up that the guide can reach it only in case of an emergency. If the store-room is to be a part of the same building, make the kitchen three or four feet longer. If separate quarters are provided for the keeping of ice, food, and other stores, it will be found wiser to put up a building six or seven feet square, rather than a mere cup-

board. The storehouse, in any case, should have a
cellar; and if the floor is boarded, this may be covered by a trap-door.

Fifth.—The proximity of the hotel makes unnecessary the laying-in of a large stock of provisions;
but on many accounts it is advantageous to buy the
staple articles of food in considerable quantities.
Flour, oatmeal, hominy, canned vegetables, potatoes,
butter, eggs, sugar, tea, coffee, and whatever else is
needed, may be bought at the hotel, much or little,
as is desired; also beef and mutton, ham and pork—
for the guide will be unhappy without the latter.
For milk it will be best to look to the nearest year-
round inhabitant who keeps a cow. From a similar
source eggs and butter may be obtained. The country is too bleak, and the soil too sandy, for the production of early spring vegetables, but, still, string
beans, green peas, sweet corn, squashes, beets, onions
and turnips, with now and then a cucumber and
musk-melon, may all be had in good time. Wild
strawberries and blueberries are plentiful. Tomatoes
rarely ripen, so that the canned article must be sub-
stituted. A week's rations will be all sufficient to
take into camp at the outset.

Sixth.—The regular guide furnishes his own boat;
but in the case of a man who is hired to take charge
of a permanent camp, he may or may not be the possessor of this indispensable accompaniment. All
other things equal, the man with a boat is much to
be preferred to the man without one. If, however,
the camper-out sees fit, he may engage a boat for the

season from the hotel, or he may buy one outright. For the other absolutely necessary things—stoves, boards for the bark building and floors, nails, mattresses, bedding, crockery, and cooking utensils, a mosquito-netting, candles—the novitiate need only make known his wants to the clerk of the hotel and all will be provided.

When the foregoing steps have been taken, the invalid will be prepared to move into camp.   As for enlarging and beautifying his primitive quarters, that will be a task to afford pleasant occupation after he has taken possession.   What has already been pointed out will be quite sufficient for him to begin the experiment comfortably and auspiciously.

CHAPTER V.

MAKING A CAMP ATTRACTIVE.

At the outset of camp life, assuming that the invalid has never tried it before, there will be, of necessity, some drawbacks and disappointments. Perhaps the weather will be cold or stormy, making it imperative to hug the stove the day through. Or perhaps the guide's manner of preparing food will prove unsatisfactory, thereby making the food itself seemingly of poor quality. Or perhaps a high wind will come up at night and roar through the trees with a dismal sound, and shake the tent with such violence that the occupant will believe his frail structure is about to be blown to atoms. Or perhaps the excitement attendant upon arranging the camp, added to the strangeness of the life, will temporarily prostrate the patient and cause the bad symptoms to display themselves with renewed virulence. Under any or all of these discomforting conditions, it must be the one great aim of the invalid not to grow discouraged. A fortnight, a month, two months may pass, and still no perceptible results of the new mode of life can be perceived. And still it is the health-seeker's one chance, to hold to the faith which first inspired him to make the experiment.

When Nature is called in as a physician, she is often disheartingly slow in her process and cure. She has none of Dr. Lumbo's liniment in her pharmacopœia. She exacts unquestioning belief in her powers, and a patience which endures with the duration of life. The experimenter in the wilderness has been in the grip of grim disease for months—for years, possibly. For months, for years, he has been breathing in the poisoned air of crowded cities and unventilated rooms. Slowly, very slowly, as the walls of the dungeon closed in, inch by inch, on the wretched prisoner, until the great apartment had become but a tomb, so the hand of disease has closed upon its victim. And this terrible grip in a day, nor a month, cannot be loosened. Perhaps it never can be loosened; but if at all, only by that slow process of Nature which prints the delicate fern upon the solid rock. That wondrously fine tissue of the lungs has been torn and wasted by the racking cough. If this waste is to be checked, it must be a work of patient labor. So, if the experiment of pure air is to be tried at all, it should be undertaken with the firm resolve to give it a full and fair trial. Otherwise, the consumptive would better keep out of the wilderness altogether.

If he has the pluck to withstand the first few discouragements which will be pretty sure to fall to his lot, the invalid will very soon discover many things about camp life which make it in the end decidedly pleasant. It is somewhat of a gift, and not wholly a virtue to be acquired, for one to adapt himself easily

3

to his surroundings. Still, will-power has something to do with making one contented. If the patient is strong enough to interest himself in the work of improving the camp, he is to be counted fortunate. Naturally, a person will take more or less pride in fitting up attractively quarters he is to occupy for a considerable period, and where the means for doing this are so abundantly furnished as in the woods, the work may be prosecuted with very gratifying results. Our suppositious invalid has thus far provided himself only with what may be termed the indispensable adjuncts of camp life. He may now, with equal pleasure and profit, devote himself to the procurement of the luxuries possible in the wilderness. The thousand and one little conveniences with which he may surround himself will tend in no small measure to make his new life attractive.

Nothing can be prettier in their way than the bark buildings to which reference has been made. One or two of these, in addition to the kitchen and storehouse, can easily be erected and serviceably used. Whatever the virtues lacking in the average Adirondack guide, mechanical ingenuity is certainly not among them. He is quick in expedients, and handles the hammer and saw like a skilful carpenter. So the bark buildings, as well as the other contrivances which may be mentioned, can be had with small outlay of time and money. One of these cabin-like structures may be fitted up as a dining-room, to be used in stormy weather or when it is too cold to eat out-of-doors. Then, an open arbor, with the roof of bark covered, is both ornamental and useful. There, in pleasant weather, the meals may be served, a stationary table being set up under the roof. If the camper-out is given to hunting and fishing, a small bark building can be utilized for the storage of guns and fishing-tackle. The guide's quarters may be either of bark or canvas, and he may be left to furnish them for himself.

A boat-landing can be readily constructed by projecting two or three heavy logs into the water and covering these with planks. It is a good thing, too, to have some sort of structure in which to store the boat when not in use. The all-serviceable bark may be used for this purpose, and the boat-house can be made an ornamental gateway to the camp. The small spruce-trees, which almost everywhere in the region are to be found in abundance, furnish precisely the material wanted for the manufacture of rustic chairs and benches. The ingenuity of the guide may be counted upon for the construction of almost every piece of furniture needful. That is, he can build chairs, tables, a lounge and bedstead ; and all these can be made not only comfortable, but tasteful, and in keeping with the surroundings. It will be seen, therefore, that there is no need to supply one's self beforehand with such articles as have been enumerated.

The work of improving and beautifying a camp may be continued indefinitely, for something will suggest itself daily, which, when done, will add to the comfort or pleasure of the life. Of course, no fixed rules can be laid down for the details of this work, since the location of the ground and individual taste must determine how to proceed. It may not be out of place, however, to sketch with some min-uteness one camp which has had an existence other than that on paper. This view, let it be remembered, is taken toward the end of the camping-out season, and after a four months' occupancy of the premises. Some idea of its situation and general appearance has already been given in these pages, but the Camp Lou of October was a very different place from the Camp Lou of June.

Standing, as has been said, on a bluff, which stretches, peninsula-like, into the clear waters of Os-good Pond, the natural advantages of the spot for the purpose desired could not well be surpassed. Almost always a cool breeze sweeps across the lake, making the air, even in the hottest days, deliciously cool. Whichever way the eye turns, it rests upon a scene of singular beauty. The densely-wooded shore across the lake rises darkly against the blue of the more distant mountains. Nowhere within the whole range of vision is there aught to be seen to mar the face of Nature by the suggestion of man's laborious toil. Not a house nor barn nor fence nor foot of cultivated soil. Nothing but the sentinel pines, and all the fragrant family of evergreens, the blue moun-tains, the clear, transparent lake, and the over-arch-ing sky. As you climb the gradual ascent which leads from the boat-landing, your feet press down a carpet of moss which grows luxuriantly on all sides. Besides this, the sandy earth is strewn with the dried pine-needles and the stubby partridge-grass, while here and there sprouts a blueberry bush, or a cluster of plume-like ferns.

Facing the lake, and in a line with the precipitous bank, stand the bark buildings and the canvas tent which collectively make up the camp. First in order comes the cabin. Its framework of spruce poles and boards is covered with wide strips of bark. The interior measures but ten feet by eight, while the porch in front, over which the roof projects, adds six feet to its length. Both the interior and porch are floored with planks, while a rustic seat outside gives an inviting appearance to the little house. The cabin is waterproof, or at all events so nearly so that the rain is not to be feared. It has its window, door, and stove, and is altogether a snug place. Within may be found a lounge, shelves containing books and magazines, a rifle hanging on the wall, chairs, and a table. In the cool autumnal days, this cabin serves as a dining-room, while in the heat of summer it affords a cool retreat for a midday nap. Next to the cabin, and a dozen or more feet beyond it, is the tent. This measures thirteen feet by twelve. The board floor is partly covered with rugs, while the open stove rests on a stone fireplace. The furniture of the tent, albeit mostly home-made, is comfortable and designed for use. There is a bed, quite as inviting as one finds in his own room. A writing-table, a set of shelves, a bookcase, a washstand, two easy chairs and a trunk, transformed into an ottoman, complete the equipments. Beyond the tent, in line with it, are

two more bark buildings, the first the kitchen and
the second the storehouse. Still further on and
nearer the bank is an open arbor, densely shaded by
spruce-trees. Then there are the guide's quarters,
and, here and there, under the branches of the trees,
rustic benches and chairs.

The stretch of level ground on which Camp Lou
is built, cost no little labor to prepare; for, originally, the earth was uneven and disfigured by the
stumps of fallen pines which may have gone down in
a forgotten forest fire. Young spruces have been set
out at various points, and gravel walks connect the
several buildings. Taken as a whole, although the
adornments are of a simple, and by no means expensive nature, the spot is attractive to the eye, and
the conveniences sufficient to make camp life a
pleasure rather than hardship.

It will be very quickly discovered by the new-
comer, that man's resemblance to the parrot is quite
as strongly developed here in the wilderness as in
the centres of civilization. The second camper-out
imitates the one who went before him, and the last
one follows pretty closely the footsteps of all who
have preceded. Another name for this imitative
faculty is fashion—and there is a prevailing fashion
even in the construction of camps. Precisely what
that is may be best learned from the guides who have
their own ideas as to how things ought to be done.
The camper-out will sometimes do better to be gov-
erned by his own judgment than by that of others.
Of course, the size of a camp should be regulated by

the number of persons it is intended to accommodate.
Its adornments will perhaps be determined by the
purse of the builder. Given the necessary equipments, and the ordinary work of a camp for two people can be satisfactorily done by one good man. If,
however, one wishes to make more of a display, half
a dozen guides—it will be remembered that this
word is used simply as a convenient way of designat-
ing those native and to the wilderness born—may be
given employment. Precisely the same rule can be
applied to the camp as to the private house, and the
domestic economy of one bears a strong resemblance
to the other. If rich enough to afford it, the patient
in the wilderness may have his valet, his cook, his
butler, his coachman, and his retinue of attendants all
as devoted as valets, cooks, butlers, and coachmen
ever were or will be. But if too poor to surround
himself with these auxiliaries, he may still live, and
live comfortably, with a single competent attendant.

Among the minor things which it will be well to
look after closely when fitting up a camp, are the
floors, especially in the tent, the stoves, and the
roofs of the bark buildings. The fact seems a little
odd, but it is none the less a fact, that in the very
heart of a lumber-growing country, lumber is unusually difficult to obtain. For the most part unplaned,
and generally unseasoned, planks are used in the construction of a camp. These serve well enough for a
majority of purposes, but when it comes to the floor-
ing of the tent, well-seasoned, matched boards, and
no others, should be used. This is of much import-

ance, for the reason that the rougher timber warps
and shrinks under the action of the weather, so that
when the colder days of autumn come around, the
floor is filled with wide crevices through which the
wind blows up uncomfortably cold.   It need hardly
be said that this is a condition of things which the
invalid should avoid.   With regard to the stoves, it
is to be remembered that whatever the season of the
year, or whatever the altitude of the mercury, no
health-seeker should think of going into camp without providing his tent with some sort of heating ap-
paratus.   Even if the days are scorchingly hot, there
is pretty sure to come a time in the twenty-four hours
when the air grows chilly; and it is always safe,
moreover, to count on some stormy days, even in
midsummer, when a fire is most acceptable.   The
necessity of making the roofs of the bark buildings
as nearly water-proof as may be, will be apparent to
all.   This can much better be accomplished when
the building is first constructed, than afterwards by
attempting to calk up the crevices.   If the boards
which support the bark on the roof be placed not
more than a foot apart, and the bark itself be lapped
over, shingle-fashion, and closely nailed, there will
be little to fear from the rain.

'   If the first season of camp life justifies the patient
in looking forward to a second trial of it, it may be a
good thing to have an ice-house built in the autumn
and stored with ice during the winter.   This may be
done with little trouble and expense.   Two or three
tons are enough to last through the camping-out

period, and besides saving the labor of bringing the
ice from the hotel, its place of storage forms a capi-
tal refrigerator for keeping supplies through the hot
weather.

The land about the St. Regis region is for the
most part private property. It is held in immense
tracts by individual owners. The right to the ground
is not, therefore, a legal one, with the camper-out.
But so long as a proper regard is shown for the pres-
ervation of the property, and care taken not to ma-
liciously injure the woodland, nobody need fear dis-
possession.

3*

CHAPTER VI.

CAMP LIFE AS AN INVALID FINDS IT.

GIVEN a fishing-rod and a rifle, as central figures; a mountain lake, flashing in the sunlight; fragrant forests of mighty pines, through which the timid deer runs affrighted at the hounds' ominous bark; hours of sweet idleness and delicious communion with nature, and, with all, a background of robust health, of high spirits, of absolute freedom from gnawing anxiety; given all these, and it is not a very difficult task to paint an attractive picture of camp life. But where these happy conditions are in many essential respects lacking; where the camp is not an Eden of a week for the tasting of sport, but the sanitarium of a season for the getting of health, and, above all, where the camper-out himself cannot cut loose from the thraldom of disease, nor know the keen pleasure of the rod and gun, then to invest camp life with anything of a charm is a more perplexing undertaking

It seems to have been assumed by all whose enthusiasm has prompted them to write and publish their experiences in the Adirondacks, that everybody is born into the world with a yearning for out-of-door

sport. Perhaps there is a large foundation in fact
for this assumption. Still it must be confessed that
now and then some wretched barbarian comes to the
surface who finds no enjoyment in a gun—no æs-
thetic delight in a fly-rod. Luckily this particular
specimen of the barbarian is rare, as are the people
who do not eat strawberries or relish oysters. But a
more numerous class of those who may hereafter seek
the wilderness as health-hunters only, will be found
composed of invalids, whose physical weakness, and
not natural inclination, will shut them off from the
enjoyment of the rod and gun. To these, more especially, this chapter will address itself, with a view
to indicating the camp life of an invalid.

It cannot be denied that this life is monotonous.
The days come and go with so little to distinguish
one from another, except it be the variable mood of
the weather, that one is really in danger of losing
track of time as completely as did Robinson Crusoe.
In densely-settled places—in the bustle of great cities—every day in the week gets to have a character
peculiar to itself. Nobody could mistake Saturday
in Central Park any more than he could Sunday at
Manhattan Beach. What thrifty New England housewife would wash on any day save Monday, or iron on
any day save Tuesday? What orthodox boarding-
house would omit to mark Friday with a fish? But
here, in the heart of the vast wilderness, there is no
Monday nor Tuesday, and only a very faint impression of Sunday. The fish sign would make Friday
of pretty much all days, while the unbroken stillness

gives seven old Puritan Sundays to every week. Take
away the ability to hunt or cast a fly, and there is
really nothing left to the camper-out in the way of
circumstantial recreation. He must devise his own
amusements, and find contentment in what, under
other conditions, would perhaps seem tame and in-
sipid. He will have always the gracious companionship of Nature—but that is something at once so
subtle and exalted, that all mankind are not permitted to enjoy it.

The camp life of an invalid will be pleasant just
in proportion to the resources within himself for
making it so. If long accustomed to find recreation
in excitement, in society, in the stimulus of city attractions, then, naturally, the seclusion and isolation
of the camp will be wearisome in the extreme. Not
a few of those who have already made the experiment of the wilderness cure have found this temporary banishment so irksome, that they have voluntarily thrown up the chance of recovering health, and
gone back to die within hearing of the gay world's
laugh. For this very reason it has seemed proper
to impress upon those who may contemplate a trial
of the Adirondacks, the necessity of preparing for all
such discomforts as they will really be called upon to
encounter. If this little book were the product of a
physician's brain, it would not be likely to deal with
the question of cure in this unscientific manner. The
medical authorities, who decree that castor oil is
sometimes a needed remedy, do not stop to discuss
the probability of the pinafored-patient's objecting

to the dose. With even better grounds, it might be assumed that the person of mature years, who is fighting a desperate disease, and who, unlike the youngster doomed to castor oil, is intelligent enough to understand that the oil is for his good only, would not hesitate to make any sacrifice of mere temporary physical comfort for the sake of ultimate recovery. And yet, limited as has been the writer's observation in this matter, it has still served to convince him that the whiskered phthisical patient is often quite as obstinate as the small boy sentenced to castor oil. Moreover, those things which are counted the veriest trifles by the strong and able-bodied, assume often an importance in the eyes of the confirmed invalid which would be ridiculous were it not seriously connected with his chances of recovery. It may so happen that an unfortunate selection of a guide will determine a patient to abandon the wilderness experiment altogether. Or, barren in resources within himself, and cut off from long-accustomed associations, he may find the quiet monotony of camp life unendurable; and, in a moment of feverish longing for the bustling city, he may hasten home, thus throwing to the winds his last hope of restored health.

The three degrees of comfort attainable in the camp of the invalid may be thus formulated: First, if the patient is in the earlier stages of the disease so that he can roam about at will, and is possessed of an honest love of nature and of the hunter's or fisherman's craft, then there is no reason why he should not be in a state of superlative contentment.

Again, supposing him still strong enough to enjoy
life, and to feel a well man's interest in what is
taking place, then, even if he has no taste for the
sportsman's pursuits, his camp life may, nevertheless,
represent comparative contentment.   But if he be an
actual sufferer from the more acute phthisical symptoms, doomed to wearying inaction, and additionally
unfortunate in possessing neither a love of sport nor
a mind to grasp the beauties of nature, then it is
easy to perceive that his lot in the wilderness will be
one of positive misery.   Yet in so deplorable a condition as the last, it may be questioned whether he
would not be positively miserable anywhere.

Nothing can add so much to the attractiveness of
the invalid's camp as congenial companionship.   The
man who is so blessed by fate as to be able to bring
wife and children into the wilderness with him—
and this, as will be demonstrated later, is practicable
even to the degree of economy—has, perhaps, the
best chance for recovery, and the smallest claim to
sympathy.   If there be no wife or child, then some
one near of kin and dear to heart should, if possible,
bear the patient company.   The society, too, of the
hotel and the neighboring camps may be sought
with profit.   Nature is sometimes wonderfully helped
in the miracle of turning the consumptives watery
blood to wine by the bright presence of kindred and
friends.   It may be, of course, impossible in all
cases for the invalid to be thus attended, but companionship should be counted by no means an unimportant element in the wilderness experiment.

After all, the thing which is pretty sure to do most toward making the sick man contented is the consciousness that he is gaining health, even if it be by inches. To a greater degree than any other method of cure which the doctors have advocated this camping-out tends to turn a man's thoughts away from his own condition. That is no small thing itself. One cannot live very long in St. Augustine or Santa Barbara, an invalid himself, without daily contact with those suffering from the same malady, and seeking the same end by precisely the same measures. That end has not been reached often enough to make the subject an encouraging one for conversation. And yet a dozen invalids thrown together will inevitably turn to their ills as the one theme in which there is unanimous interest. Still worse, on this account, is any regular sanitarium, where the constant society of those similarly afflicted must be, as it always has been, a serious drawback to recovery. In the wilderness camp the patient is effectually removed from all these unfavorable conditions. Around and about him on every side, are the evidences of vigorous life. Life in the grand old pines, in the whispering poplar, in the tough-fibred tamarack; life in the tapping of the woodpecker, in the drum of the partridge, in the whistle of the robin; life in the startled deer, as it leaps affrighted into the dense underbrush, and in the squirrel as he springs nimbly from branch to branch; life in the placid lakes and laughing stream, in the fresh breezes that blow across the land, in sky and earth and water—everywhere life. And so the

shadow of the great destroyer is swallowed up in
the sunlight and beauty and grandeur of nature.

Then, too, this isolation which the camp affords is
not allied to that sense of loneliness which attends
the invalid who seeks more remote resorts. I address myself now, of course, to those who live in the
Eastern and Middle States, for from this vast region
thousands of health-seekers have gone forth in the
past, journeying to far-away places, nor ever bethink-
ing them of the rare virtues of this forest which
lies, as it were, at their doors. Probably every physician of much experience has had occasion to note
the ill effects which frequently attend this removal
from home and friends. There is a kind of heart
yearning—call it homesickness, if you please—which
takes hold of a sick man banished to unfamiliar places, too strong to be resisted. Now, while an Adirondack camp may seem cut off from the busy world
as completely as a South Pacific island, yet the invalid knows that in fact he is not very far away from
his home. He knows that the journey back is no
very great undertaking. In short, he knows that he
can put an end to his voluntary banishment to-mor-
row, if he chooses. And that gives him courage to
remain to-day. So far as the writer's own case is
concerned, this sense of freedom to do as he pleased
went a good way toward making camp life endurable.

Even a more important consideration than that of
contentment, is the relative cost of the wilderness
cure as compared with that of living in the places
which have heretofore been regarded as the consump-

tive's hope. This matter of money has nothing to do with the theory of therapeutic measures, but, unfortunately, it has a great deal to do with the practice of them. Man is presumed to value his life beyond any worldly possession. To the hard alternative of surrendering a remunerative position and expending his last dollar, or yielding up his life, a vast majority of mankind would unhesitatingly accept the former. But what is one to do if he has no treasure to give in lieu of his life? What is the clerk, dependent on his meagre wages, to answer when the physician tells him that he must go to the South of France or Lower California, if he does not want to die within six months? As well recommend him to go to the moon; and the more certain the belief that the impossible trip would restore him to health and strength, the more bitter his cup, as he reflects on the utter inability of any man to reach the moon. But even the clerk can reach this wilderness and pitch his tent, and try the experiment which may give him a new lease of life.

If the camp life of the invalid is monotonous, it is not, as has already been indicated, a life of either privation or hardship. The sick man gets up in the morning when he feels like it—say nine o'clock. He finds at hand all the conveniences for making a toilet, and when he steps from the tent into the crisp, fresh air, he ought to be hungry and thankful. A breakfast, as good as any man can reasonably expect, is ready, steaming hot. Excellent butter, smoking muffins, fragrant coffee, and eggs which no man ever saw longer

ago than yesterday; a dish of dainty trout, now
crisply fried in cracker-crumbs, but two hours ago
jumping at flies in the water; baked or fried potatoes, with a leaf of fresh salad; milk that produces
more cream to the square inch than the city-restau-
rant fluid does to the acre; and with all this, the
inevitable wheat-cake, hot from the griddle, served
with a generous supply of maple-syrup. It is well
on to ten o'clock when the breakfast is over. Then,
if the day be warm and fair, the camper-out may
lounge under the trees and read the daily papers—a
day or two old, to be sure, but fresh enough up here.
Or he may take a turn on the lake, and try his hand
at fishing. Somewhere about one o'clock he is expected to grapple with a lunch of cold beef or chicken
or mutton, bread and butter, milk, fruit, and cake.
Then he may sleep or read or write or philosophize,
or wander off to explore the surrounding forests—
do anything, in short, that his fancy dictates. At
six o'clock he sits down to a dinner which, if not rel-
ished, will be the fault of the eater only. Roast venison or lamb, green corn, tomatoes, potatoes, cucum-
bers, squash and beets, with a tempting entree or
two, in the shape of frogs' legs or game, salad, and a
blueberry pudding, not lacking the brandy-sauce—
there is his menu. After that a cigar and an hour
about a roaring camp-fire; or, later in the season, a
fire within the tent, the canvas flaps cozily drawn,
the student-lamp lighted, a good book, or a game at
chess, backgammon or cards at his preference. Then
bed.

The domestic economy of the camp is generally in-trusted to the guide; and, if he be the right sort of a man, this method saves considerable trouble. If, however, a more direct supervision of affairs becomes desirable, there is no reason why it cannot be exercised.   Supposing the camp to contain but two persons, the invalid and his companion, and supposing, further, that the money question cannot be eliminated from the wilderness experiment, then one competent guide should be counted as sufficient for all the work, for the daily routine labors in a permanent camp are neither very burdensome nor very numerous. The chief difficulty is to find a really good man who takes kindly to this sort of life.   Very many of them prefer the much harder task of "guiding" proper, with its attendant excitement and nomadic charm. And perhaps this is not to be wondered at; for their lives are monotonous enough through the greater portion of the year to make them keenly appreciative of the company of pleasure-seeking sportsmen.   Then, too, many of them feel, and rightly, that they are capable of something better than washing dishes and making beds.   There is, indeed, no reason why the ordinary work of the invalid's camp should not be performed by a woman.   The duties would not be unlike those of the average hired girl, in the average city house.   To cook the food would be her chief task.   Add to the woman a strong, active boy to chop wood, draw water, and run errands, and the domestic machinery of a camp could certainly be kept in harmonious motion.   Not that the services of a guide are not desirable always, and indispensable where the invalid intends to devote himself to hunting or fishing; but the suggestion is made for the benefit of those who may care nothing for the latter pursuits, and who are compelled to economize in order to make the experiment at all.

Depending largely upon the hotel for supplies, as most of the permanent camps do, it is customary to send over daily for the mail, and such stores as may be needed. This regular receiving of the mail marks a bright hour in the day. The incentive of getting it may also lead the patient, when his strength shall have so far returned as to warrant it, to walk over to the hotel, and thus get an hour's tramp equally pleasant and beneficial.

Although the experiment has never, I believe, been made, there is certainly no reason why a person desiring to avoid the delay or trouble of fitting up a camp, might not pitch a tent in the woods surrounding "Paul" Smith's, and take his meals at the hotel, while sleeping under canvas. This would give him the benefit of the great end sought—the constant breathing in of pure air—and at the same time it would assure him an excellent table. It would hardly do to recommend the plan on the score of economy, however, as it would probably prove more expensive than the full-fledged camp.

Nobody should attempt a prolonged residence in this wilderness without that steadfast friend and faithful companion—a dog. The Adirondack spaniel, which is, perhaps, the most common breed here, is pos-

sessed of a degree of intelligence, docility, and good
nature which raise him to the rank of the princes of
his kind.   He is not often pretty to the eye, nor would
he, as a rule, pass muster under the close scrutiny of a
dog-fancier; but if not pretty, he is good, and if
lacking in "points," he is rich in affection.   He takes
to partridges as naturally as the terrier to rats, and
he develops often into an acute and sagacious hunter.
His unvarying mildness is perhaps due, in part, to
his diet—for the Adirondack dog gets very little
meat.   There is also the deer-hound, excellent in his
special line of work, but less companionable than the
spaniel.   Many an hour which would otherwise drag
wearily in camp, may be pleasantly passed in canine
company. ˙Your dog never burdens you with long
stories or impertinent inquiries.   He never has a sure
cure for your cough, which he insists upon your trying.   He is never moody nor out of sorts, nor averse
to a frolic.   In short, he is tip-top company for a
sick man.

The camp may also afford refuge for live chickens,
and it might even be practicable to keep a cow. Dr.
Trudeau has a high opinion of the nutritive qualities
of milk, and has accustomed himself to take eight or
ten glasses through the day.

Altogether the camp life of the invalid ought to
be made as bright, as cheerful, and as comfortable
as the circumstances of the place will admit. If
sometimes the days drag monotonously—and they
will—let it be kept steadily in mind that if the experiment is worth making at all, it is worth making

well and thoroughly. And if weeks, and even months, should pass, bringing little of that restored strength which was promised, then let this solacing reflection arise, that in nearly every instance where the case has been serious, the patient has been called upon thus similarly to put his faith to the test, but that in the end the wilderness has wrought a cure which has sometimes seemed little less than a miracle.

CHAPTER VII.

THE proposition to spend a winter in the Adirondack wilderness, when first made to a consumptive invalid, shivering even in the May temperature of New York City, seemed grotesquely absurd. Most of us have long been taught to look upon mild climate as a prime requisite in the cure of weak lungs. To accept, in place of this orthodox creed, one diametrically opposed thereto, and to voluntarily go in search of what heretofore we had conscientiously run away from, was like stumbling upon a new Galileo, with a new dogma to shake fixed faith and disarrange the stars themselves.

And yet this experiment of sending pulmonary patients to winter in a cold region is by no means new or untried. The virtues of the Alps in this matter have been put to the test for many years, and with results that abundantly justify the theory. In an untechnical, but interesting, paper, published some two or three years ago in the *Fortnightly Review*, and entitled "Davos in Winter," many facts are given which bear so directly on the subject in hand, that I may be pardoned for reproducing some brief

extracts therefrom. The writer tells us that a German
physician of repute, himself far gone in consumption,
determined in 1865 to try whether high Alpine air
was really a cure for serious lung disease. In spite
of having to rough it more than invalids find safe
and pleasant, the doctor derived so much benefit from
his first visit that he persevered and ultimately recovered his health. The result is that Doctor Unger
and his fellow-workers have transformed Davos from
a mere mountain village into a health-station fre-
quented by nearly one thousand invalids who passed
the winter with every comfort of good accommodation, excellent food, and not a few amusements.
Continuing, the writer in the *Review* says: "The
method of cure is very simple. After a minute personal examination of the ordinary kind, your physician tells you to give up medicines, and to sit warmly
clothed in the sun as long as it is shining, to eat as
much as possible, to drink a fair quantity of Valtel-
line wine, and not to take any exercise. He comes
at first to see you every day, and soon forms a more
definite opinion of your capacity and constitution.
Then, little by little, he allows you to walk; at first
upon the level, next up-hill, until the daily walks
begin to occupy from four to five hours. The one
thing relied upon is air. To inhale the maximum
quantity of the pure mountain air, and to imbibe the
maximum quantity of the keen mountain sunlight,
is the *sine quâ non*. Every thing else—milk-drink-
ing, douches, baths, friction, counter-irritant appli-
cations, and so forth—is subsidiary. Medicine is very

rarely used; and yet the physicians are not pedan-
tic in their dislike of drugs. They only find by long
experience that they can get on better without medicine. Therefore they do not use it except in cases
where their observation shows that it is needed. And
certainly they are justified by the result. The worst
symptoms of pulmonary sickness—fever, restless
nights, cough, blood-spitting, and expectoration—
gradually subside by merely living and breathing.
The appetite returns, and the power of taking exercise is wonderfully increased. When I came to Davos, for example, at the beginning of last August, I
could not climb two pairs of stairs without the greatest discomfort. At the end of September I was able
to walk one thousand feet up hill without pain and
without fear of hemorrhage. This progress was maintained throughout the winter.; and when I left Davos,
in April, the physician could confirm my own sensa-
tion that the lung, which had been seriously injured,
was comparatively sound again, and that its wound
had been healed. Of course I do not mean that the
impossible had been achieved, or, in other words,
that what had ceased to be organic had been recom-
posed for me, but that the disease had been arrested
by a natural process of contraction."

All that the writer here claims for the little Alpine
village may be applied with equal force to the St.
Regis country. If the elevation of the latter is much
less than that of the former, the purity of the atmosphere, the abundance of sunlight, the complete absence of anything like dampness, and the almost

4

magical results of the climate, are all as characteristic
of the Adirondack wilderness as of Davos. Here, as
there, the worst symptoms of pulmonary complaints
subside by merely living and breathing. Here, as
there, the appetite returns, and the progress of the
disease is arrested. But, whereas in Davos, the patient finds himself forced to combat the evil influences attending a sanitarium, to which reference
has already been made in these pages, in the wilderness he may utterly avoid contact with people afflicted like himself; and, whereas, to a thousand
Americans upon whom consumption has laid its
skeleton hand, the long journey to the Alps would be
as impossible as a tour around the world, this experiment of the wilderness may be made—and made with
small outlay and little discomfort. So I hope it will
not be charged to the overenthusiasm of the writer
if he claims even greater virtues for the Adirondacks
than others may for Davos.

Dividing the year into the two seasons of camp
life and house life, the former, although necessarily
varying somewhat in length, may be set down as
covering at its maximum five months. It will very
seldom be found safe to get into camp before the
first of June; nor is it, as a rule, desirable to remain
later than the middle of October. These remaining
seven months, then, constitute the winter season in
the wilderness—that is, the season of house life. By
this phrase, however, is not meant a life of indoor
indolence. In winter, not less than summer, the
great end sought after is to breathe all the pure air

possible, and to keep out-of-doors as much of the time as the condition of the patient warrants.

Saranac Lake, which is something of a town for the backwoods, and which lies on the Saranac River, about thirteen miles from "Paul" Smith's, and six from Bloomingdale, has heretofore been the point to which invalids remaining through the winter have turned most often. It may be explained that Saranac Lake is here applied not to the body of water bearing that name, but to the post-office; and the post-office, with the aid of weak lungs, has resulted in building up a diminutive village. A few of the winter health-seekers have remained at the St. Regis Lake House, whenever that comfortable inn has been kept open. During the past winter the house was closed to boarders. This sent the majority of invalids to Saranac. The writer, for reasons which will hereafter be explained, preferred to take up his abode in the town of Brighton, Franklin County, on the main road which leads from Bloomingdale to "Paul" Smith's. So far as the climatic benefits are concerned, it is really a matter of no consequence whether the invalid spends the winter at St. Regis Lake, Bloomingdale, or Saranac. I should not presume to make this statement except on the authority of a physician who has passed a number of winters in the immediate neighborhood referred to, and whose opinion is entitled to the highest respect.

To those who depend largely upon society for recreation, and who are without other resources of con-

tentment, Saranac Lake may be recommended as the
most desirable spot in which to pass the winter.
Not that the village offers other than a very mild
type of excitement, but in the backwoods we must
measure attractions in a liberal spirit. By chance,
or otherwise, Dr. Trudeau hit upon the village as the
place for spending his first winter in the wilderness,
and since that time many others have followed his
example. The result is that a comfortable boarding-
house, known as the Berkley, has been fitted up with
a special view to the accommodation of invalids.
There are also a number of smaller houses where
good board may be obtained at reasonable rates.
The Saranac Lake House, called by everybody here
Martin's, stands at the northern extremity of the little lake of the same name, a mile or so from the village. Next to "Paul" Smith's, Martin's is perhaps
the best-known inn anywhere in the wilderness. It
has not, I believe, heretofore been kept open through
the winter, but board could probably be obtained there
if one chose to apply for it. Saranac gets its daily
mail, enjoys telegraphic communication, and is connected by stage with Elizabethtown, as well as Ausable Forks. Besides these advantages, a sufficient
number of health-seekers were to be found there last
winter to constitute a little social coterie. There is an
Episcopal church, regularly supplied with a clergy-
man, while the Methodists worship in the school-
house. The post-office holds its treasures in a store,
where letters and groceries are meted out together.

What to others would perhaps seem an attraction,

to the writer appeared as the one drawback in connection with Saranac. It was to rid himself of the companionship of other invalids, agreeable as that companionship might be, invalidism apart, that he avoided the place of more common resort, and found a winter home with a farmer-guide in Brighton.

If the camp life of an invalid is of necessity somewhat monotonous, his winter life in these woods must be even more so. And yet there is so much to compensate for the self-imposed exile, that the winter, to my thinking, is fraught with greater charms than the summer. Others, I know, will not agree with me in this respect; but all who make the experiment will surely discover that wintering in the wilderness is a far pleasanter process of cure than they pictured it in fancy. A measure of monotony is conceded; but monotony is productive of a methodical manner of life—of regularity of habits which the doctors praise and all the sage saws of the world seek to inculcate. I am forced to admit that the first winter I spent in the Adirondacks failed miserably to sustain its reputation for evenness of temperature and extreme cold. This, however, must be attributed to the exceptional character of that season the country over. As a rule, the winter months here will be found dry, bracing, and remarkably free from thaws. As a rule, also, to which the winter of 1879–80 afforded a striking exception, snow falls in great abundance, and three or four months of continuous sleighing are counted upon with certainty. In spite of its unusual mildness, the winter we spent in the woods serves to illustrate what the cold season in the Adirondacks can do toward strengthening weak lungs.

It was early enough, certainly, when the wilderness first put on its winter robes. We broke camp in a snow-storm on November 3d, and the backwoods sovereigns, who were called upon the next day to exercise their glorious right of suffrage, drove to the polls in cutters and bob-sleds. But this premature promise of winter's arrival had melted completely away, even before the hopes of many a beaten candidate were extinguished in his heart. November gave us scarcely a taste after that of genuine winter. Throughout December there were some bright, clear days scattered at intervals; in January we saw the thermometer once or twice mark a temperature of twenty-five degrees below zero, although the month, as a whole, was unreasonably warm; while in February, bringing, as it did, more snow than the resident of New York City is likely often to see, there were times when the mercury got up to preposterously high figures, standing in the sun, once at least, above sixty. Thaws were unpleasantly frequent, and although taken as a whole, there were many days of excellent sleighing, this was so often interrupted that a carriage was more serviceable on many occasions than a sleigh. Still, in spite of these unexpected drawbacks, the climate continued to work an improvement in the writer's condition. Neither did the sudden and often extreme changes in the temperature produce any of those ill effects which almost invariably follow in other regions. With a jump of the mercury from twenty-five degrees below zero to fifty degrees above, in twenty-four hours' time, exposure to the out-of-door air was attended with no bad results. The capacity of the soil to absorb all surface moisture, even in midwinter, is certainly astonishing. The atmosphere, too, seems absolutely free from dampness, even while the snow is melting under one's feet. In short, if steady and decided improvement could be made under the exceptionally unfavorable conditions of the winter in question, then ordinarily the cold season in the Adirondacks must prove highly beneficial to weak lungs.

In sketching briefly the manner of life here in winter, the writer must draw chiefly upon his own experience. If others, like him, should regard it as desirable to search out a private boarding-place, it will be by no means difficult to accomplish that end. Along the main road, between Bloomingdale and St. Regis Lake, are scattered numerous farm-houses, in almost any one of which comfortable accommodation could probably be had. The village of Bloomingdale itself contains a good-sized inn and several dwellings of more pretentious appearance than those on the road. There are two or three stores in the place, a telegraph station, post-office, public school, and church. Certain advantages are gained if one prefers the seclusion of a private house by living on the stage road, although pleasant quarters can, no doubt, be found in many of the more remote houses. If the means of recreation through the winter months are limited, they may still serve to prevent the time from hanging heavily on the invalid's hands. In the bright, clear, sunshiny days—and a good many of these may be counted upon in the course of the season—it will be the first duty of the patient to keep as much out of doors as is practicable. If his strength justifies him in taking moderate bodily exercise, he may walk over the roads with a scene before his eyes grander than was ever yet put on canvas ; or he may strike across lots through the woods on a pair of snow-shoes, which barbarous contrivances are here indicative of civilization; or he may hunt rabbits ; and if he knows how to use his gun, he may be sure of plenty of this lively game. Should he be still too weak to safely indulge in these more violent exercises, he may ride out instead, and thereby secure to himself the benefit of the bracing air without the slightest fear of taking cold. The majority of the year-round inhabitants own horses, and it is not therefore difficult to obtain some sort of turnout. The writer found riding a more congenial form of exercise than any other, and made it a point to go out at least once a day, except in extremely stormy weather. It may not be out of place in this connection to recommend the purchase of a buffalo-skin overcoat as by far the most suitable garment for winter wear in the wilderness. These coats are inexpensive, durable, and the only things that have been discovered warm enough to protect a person riding against the cutting winds that sweep across this country.

It may not fall to the lot of all others to secure so

home-like and comfortable a boarding-place as did the writer, but it is safe to say that the health-seeker will be well provided for in his wilderness abode. In the matter of food, the resources of the country are naturally less rich in winter than summer. After the first of December few if any trout are taken, nor should there be. The period in which deer may legally be killed expires now in this State the first of December, I believe. At all events, venison is a pretty juiceless meat in midwinter, and very little of it is offered for sale in the St. Regis region. Partridges string along until January, but they lose in plumpness and flavor, and are by no means abundant. Cutting off thus trout, deer, and birds, the domestic menu of the woods reduces itself chiefly to pork and potatoes. This diet hardly meets the wants of the consumptive patient, but he will find that those who make a business of taking boarders will not expect him to subsist thereon. Our own table, which was set distinct from that of the household, was liberally supplied with beef, mutton, chickens, winter and canned vegetables, eggs, excellent bread, fresh butter, and milk. It is pleasant to speak in praise of the cooking of the Adirondack housewife, and if the experience of others coincides with the writer's, such praise will be happily justified. One thing, however, cannot share in the smallest measure in this otherwise complimentary report. If there be anything poorer in the way of meat than the average Adirondack beef, then most of us, I hope, have yet to discover it. It is tough, dry, and tasteless. If it

4*

has any mission in the world, it is to teach resignation, while it strengthens the muscles of the jaw. This unvarnished truth applies equally to all beef raised and slaughtered here. Even at the best of the hotels the best of their beef would surely be criticized in a fifteen-cent city restaurant. The fault is in the country, rather than in the people; and the deficiency can only be supplied by having good beef sent on from some point where good beef is to be had. I speak thus particularly of this matter because of the large dependence which the physicians place upon nourishing beef in the diet of the consumptive patient. For any other delicacies it will also be necessary to look to the city markets; but barring the beef, a wholesome and nutritious diet will be found in the winter boarding-house.

With pleasant indoor accommodations, an excellent table, a daily drive of two or three hours, an occasional jaunt on foot, plenty of books and newspapers, and the cheering consciousness of steady progress toward recovery, the winter life of the invalid in this remote wilderness may, after all, be counted an endurable one. If the first week or two after the breaking-up of camp should be followed by some return of the bad symptoms, it need cause no alarm. As a rule, after sleeping three or four months in a tent, any room, however well ventilated, will seem close and stifling. The lungs, long accustomed to the absolute purity of the tent air, become acutely sensitive to whatever is vitiated or foul. As a matter of fact, the atmosphere of a well-lighted, properly ventilated room in one of these wilderness houses is incomparably purer than the most imposing apartment in the finest city residence. While, therefore, the change from the tent to the bedroom may here be accompanied with some unpleasant effects, it is quite certain that this change will be far less perceptible than would the sudden transition from the wilderness house to the city home.

Among the writer's friends who shook their heads ominously over the idea of sending a sick man into the bleak woods to pass a winter, it was a common argument that if a person was compelled to spend the greater portion of the time in-doors, why not remain at home where in-door life would certainly be more attractive? These kindly advisers forget that the air within doors can never be purer than that outside. It may, and perhaps of necessity must, be less pure. If, then, the air is bad without, it will be the same air made worse within; while if pure without, it will be by so much the purer in-doors. In a word, there is no special atmosphere manufactured for house use. Shut up in a room in Water street, a person must breathe Water street air; housed in the wilderness, he still inhales none other than wilderness air. And with no noxious odors, no defective drains or gas-pipes, no miserable furnaces, no double windows to shut out the oxygen—with none of these abominations, but in place thereof, cheery wood-fires, open chimney-places, and a surrounding atmosphere of absolute purity, it must be admitted that in-door life in the Adirondacks gives the lungs something very different from the air of the average city house.

The wilderness winter, as a rule, lingers so long in the lap of spring that he leaves very little of the calendar to be reigned over by the balmier season. Often the sleighing stretches far into April, and the ice in the lakes has been known to remain until the 10th of May. This makes June very like a Long Island April. Happily, however, the transition from winter to spring is attended with very few, if any, of those sudden changes which are apt to prove so trying to weak lungs in places like New York and Boston. And this adds another to the many virtues of the Adirondack region, the more conspicuous because it is possessed by so few of the health resorts. Even our Davos enthusiast admits that the Alpine village should be deserted by the invalid with the first approach of spring. Here, all seasons seem to afford more or less benefit to the consumptive. He is not forced to fly at the approach of spring or to interrupt the slow processes of nature with the coming of the winter. To all who may be induced to try the wilderness experiment, the writer would say, and say most earnestly, that the winter residence is quite as essential as the camp life through the warmer months. Even if the latter fails to accomplish any perceptible good in the patient's condition, let him still hold fast to his faith in the cold-weather theory. The danger is, that either discouraged at the absence of the results expected, or, in more fortunate cases, made too confident by a speedy progress toward recovery, the invalid yields to a natural desire to return to home and kindred or to those pursuits which he fancies he is strong enough to follow, and so puts an end to the experiment before he has given it half a trial. An active, energetic man may look upon a year's banishment from the field of his labors as too hard a sentence; but a shorter sojourn than that, where pulmonary disease has taken any firm hold on its victim, will fail to give the wilderness cure a reasonable test. It must be winter as well as summer—perhaps two or three winters and two or three summers. A long game—but the stakes are high.

CHAPTER VIII.

MR. RICHARD GRANT WHITE has somewhere put
on record that, to his thinking, "there is nothing in
the world more charming than simple, unpretending
ignorance, nothing more respectable, nothing surer
to elicit sympathy from healthy minds." If this use
of words be not an abuse, then to find what is supremely charming, overwhelmingly respectable, and
superlatively deserving of sympathy Mr. White and
the rest of the world should come up here and min-
gle with the native inhabitants.

To the year-round resident of the wilderness the
world is bounded by Canada on the north, Plattsburg on the east, Boonville on the south, and Malone on the west. All that lies beyond this clearly
defined territory is dim, shadowy, and uncertain.
The end and aim of life is to "guide" in summer,
and "log" in winter. Nowhere else on the face of
the earth is it so easy to divide all people into classes
at once so distinct and comprehensive. Every man
must come under one of the two heads—he must be
either a guide or a sportsman. For the qualifications
of the latter, anything like previous training is un-

necessary.   The writer freely confesses that before he came into the St. Regis country he had never to his knowledge, shot off a gun in his life, except possibly the air-guns that are sometimes made a tributary means of revenue in church fairs ; he had never cast a fly, nor jointed a rod, nor told a fish story—intentionally, at any rate—he had never seen a deer save those in Central Park, while the few "strikes" he ever made on speckled trout were confined exclusively to Fulton Market.   And yet—the assertion is made with a full sense of the responsibility that may hereafter attach thereto—and yet he was not fairly in the wilderness before he made the startling discovery that he was a "sportsman."   So much for one of the grand divisions of mankind as found in the St. Regis country.   The other is far more unique and interesting.

To begin with, the nationality of these backwoodsmen is a mixed problem.   French blood mingles in at least equal proportions with American, and probably nine-tenths of all the people are descended more or less directly from Canadian ancestors.   The French of Canada is not exactly the French of Paris, but it may be said to bear about the same relation to the latter that the sardine does to the herring.   Ichthyologists classify these fishes under the same family head, but it is not very difficult to distinguish between them.   Here in the immediate St. Regis Lake region a large proportion of the inhabitants speak Canadian French with at least as much facility as they speak English.   The vastness of the country, as compared with the population, has led to such a complex intermarrying that pretty nearly everybody is either the aunt or uncle or cousin of everybody else. If the soil yields but a sorry harvest of grain, it seems at least adapted to the production of large families. A dozen children and sometimes a score grow to robust maturity in spite of all hardship and privation. That the life of these people is a hard one—that the privations they are called upon to endure are such as would drive away a less hardy or stubborn race—is not to be denied. The few acres of land that have been cleared and cultivated return at best but a meagre harvest for the most unremitting toil. Through the long winter the one industry which offers employment is the chopping and drawing of logs. Many a man is glad to swing an axe ten hours out of the twenty-four for seventy-five cents wages. Ready money is always scarce and always hoarded. Young and old live principally on pork and potatoes, with now and then a soup of dry beans or peas. Sheep thrive here fairly well, but the mutton is, as a rule, regarded too valuable a product to be used for food. The wife of the backwoodsman works even more untiringly than her husband, and in the absence of the latter often does unaided the drudgery which should be assigned only to men.

But there comes a genial ray of sunlight into the wilderness with the advent of the sportsmen. It is then that every man and boy is ready to offer his services as a guide. The guide does not grow. He bears a striking resemblance to the city barber in that he never serves an apprenticeship. The world, or at least as much of it as is shaved, long ago discovered that the barber-shop never existed which employed other than experienced " artists." It follows, therefore, that the barber, full-fledged, springs up in the night or else drops from the skies, razor in hand, and the praises of the best hair tonic in the world on his lips. Similarly comes the Adirondack guide into this barren world. He rolls, so to speak, out of his log cradle into a pair of top boots, discards the bottle for a plug of tobacco, possesses himself of a boat and a jackknife, and becomes forthwith an experienced guide. His duties are multifarious. He pulls a steady if not exactly scientific oar; he carries his boat on his shoulders from one mountain pond to another, often a distance of two or three miles; he conducts you to the spot where deer ought to be, and where sometimes they are; he fishes for you if you don't know how to fish for yourself, and breaks your new fly-rod with perfect good humor; if in camp, he cooks and chops wood and forecasts the weather with an unvarying inaccuracy which would discourage the most hopeful of meteorological prophets. It would never do to assert that the Adirondack guide is constitutionally lazy after thus particularizing his labors. True, he is forced to drag through seven or eight months of the year in waiting for the other four or five months to come around; but that is not his fault. Nor is this period of waiting by any means one of idle ease. The winter work is far more laborious and much less profitable than the summer guiding. Many of the men spend a good part of the cold season in a logger's camp, as it is called, and that is a kind of camp which offers very few attractions. It implies steady chopping from sunrise to sunset, exposure to the coldest weather, coarse fare, small wages, and no pleasanter recreation than a pipeful of tobacco in the evening. Harder even than the cutting, "skidding" (which means piling), or drawing of logs, is the driving of them down the rivers in the spring. The drivers are often drenched with water or half frozen by cold; and they run no inconsiderable risk of losing life or limb. The work pays better, however, than any other branch of the lumberman's calling.

Besides the severity of the winter work here, there is frequently no job to be had even at the small wages demanded. Last winter, for example, the lack of sleighing, without which the drawing of logs cannot be undertaken, shut out many men from the chance of earning a few needed dollars. Were it not that the cost of living is reduced to its minimum, the less thrifty inhabitants would be driven to sorry straits. Many of them are poor enough, as it is; but there is none of that acute suffering from poverty which is to be found in the cities. Oddly enough, the want of money here, while it may enhance its value as a personal possession, seems to give to the native a supreme indifference for the wealth of others. This wealth may have its existence wholly in the imagination, as much of it indeed does; but that is of small matter so long as the stock of imagination holds out. The Adirondack guide, whose uncertain income seldom reaches five hundred dollars a year, will talk to you of millions with the refreshing assurance of Colonel Sellers. He sets every man down as rich who comes into the wilderness unpursued by a deputy-sheriff. He believes that every man is a sportsman because he is rich, and that he is rich because he is a sportsman, and that he is both because he is not a St. Regis guide. There you have the pith of backwoods logic in a nutshell.

The crossing of nationalities—the uncommon congenital mixture of a French peasant and a Yankee backwoodsman—gives rise to some curious combinations in names. You may find the thoroughly Anglo-Saxon James, John, and Henry, flanked by such surnames as St. Germain, La Bountie and Robal. You may have your faith in philology sadly shaken by the discovery that Mitchell Sweeney is a Frenchman, and that Mrs. Stephen Otis cannot speak English. It is a noteworthy fact that almost without exception the French residents give no hint of their nationality in speaking English. It may not be very pure English, but it is certainly freer from provincialisms and infinitely better in its pronunciation than is the speech of the average rural New Englander.

This wilderness must be set down as a spot which puts greatness to a terribly severe test, and extinguishes notoriety with a beautiful simplicity. Edison's name is unknown, and the thrifty housewife who told me that she thought she remembered vaguely of having once heard of Henry Ward Beecher, compelled an indescribable admiration. The late Vice-President of the United States secure his claim to recognitioń, not because of the office he held, but because he lived in Malone. John Brown is not here the martyr to a great cause, but the man who bought a big tract of land in North Elba. I remember, at the time when the tempest-tossed bones of the late A. T. Stewart were rattled afresh in the public ears, Joshua La Fontaine came over to camp one day on a friendly visit. We fell to talking together, and I drew out some curious confessions from Joshua. He had lived the thirty-five years of his life wholly in the woods. He had never visited a city, nor even a village; never had ridden on a railway, nor seen a steam engine; never had been to a circus nor to school; was in doubt as to whether Plattsburg was a bigger place than New York; and was profoundly impressed by the statement that the earth is round and not flat. The mention of Plattsburg suggested the Stewart case for the double reason that, in the correspondence printed a few days before, that town had incidentally figured, and also because Plattsburg was reasonably to be considered within Joshua's geographical grasp.

"They seem to have found out where Stewart's body is, at last," said I, taking up the newspaper which contained the report.

"Yer don't say so?" said Joshua, evincing at once the keenest interest in the subject.

"Yes; and, according to the story here, it passed through Plattsburg on its way to Montreal."

"My land o' the livin', now, who'd a thought that?" rejoined Joshua, gazing meditatively at the back of his left hand while he worked the fingers as if to test their joints.

"If what the paper says is true, Judge Hilton can get the remains by the payment of two hundred and fifty thousand dollars."

"He ken, ken he? Wall, now, I'll be chewed!"

"Yes; the thieves sent on the silver plate and the piece of coffin-lining that was cut out, so there can be no question about identity."

"Jes'so! And the Jedge ken git 'em for two hundred and fifty-thousand dollars?"

"That's the sum. Seems pretty big, doesn't it— but there's money enough back, you know."

"Two hundred and fifty thousand dollars!" repeated Joshua, still studying with profound interest the back of his hand. "Wall, now, I'd never athought old Stewart left as much as that behind him!"

"Why, bless your soul, he left probably a hundred times that sum!"

"Old Jeems Stewart did?"

"Jeems? His name wasn't Jeems—it was Alexander—A. T. Stewart."

There was dead silence for half a minute, and then Joshua, finishing the inspection of his last knuckle, remarked:

"I thought yer was talking about Jeems Stewart who bought that thar mill up at Keeseville. I guess I never heared of this other one—Alexander B., did you say?"

"T.," I murmured faintly. And there ended my effort to discuss affairs of the day with Joshua La Fontaine.

Under this surface of calm indifference to all that is passing in the great world outside, there is a solid basis of content. Without this the Adirondack back-woodsman would be impossible. His ignorance, after all, is superficial; his wisdom is deep-rooted and practical. He may not be able to write his name, but he can read with unerring accuracy the chirography of nature. He may not know his letters, but he never trips on the alphabet of forest lore. He finds himself born to a lot of privation and hardship. Instead of repining over this, or vainly coveting the fortune of the more prosperous, he sets to work man-fully to make the best of his surroundings. In an exceptional degree he is thrifty, saving, and indus-trious. Not a few of the men in the St. Regis country have, by the dint of unflagging toil, amassed a competence. They recognize, apparently by some intuitive wisdom, that while the lines of their life here are not cast in easy places, still it is here that they can best fight the battle for bread. They have no desire to throw themselves into the vortex of city life, nor are they often led away by the *ignis fatuus* of the indefinite West. In this respect, and especially among the young men, the prevailing characteristic of the year-round inhabitant is peculiar. In almost every farming region, the dream of the younger gen-eration is to break loose from home moorings, and cast their fortune upon the untried sea of the world outside. Here, on the contrary, this ambition for a larger field of action—this craving to see and know something of the busy world we inhabit—seems to be utterly lacking. If content be indeed another name for happiness, the dwellers in the wilderness ought to be supremely happy. The green earth over, there certainly could be found no better spot in which temporarily to plant a college sophomore or a rural Congressman. The small vanities and pretensions of a man will be taken out of him here with much the same jerky suddenness that a fish is taken out of the water. He may be great in a town, great in a State, great even in a nation; he will be small as a midge here unless he can cast a scientific fly, or hit a buck at a hundred yards.

Hard-working, truthful, sober, book-ignorant, nature-wise—this is the general character of these backwoods dwellers. And yet you cannot bunch these men and label them with any one ticket. Here, as elsewhere, the good and the bad may be found ; and under a crust of laziness and saleratus I have discovered many a brave, patient, and heroic nature— men like the trees they have grown up among, sturdy and upright as the grand old pine, yet as full of the juices of humanity as the maple is full of sap in spring.

CHAPTER IX.

To Professor Alfred L. Loomis, of New York City, belongs, in a very large degree, the honor of awakening in the medical profession a lively interest in the curative powers of the Adirondacks. A paper of his on this subject was read before The Medical Society of the State of New York in 1879, and afterward printed in the *Medical Record*. That paper must stand as the excuse for this little book. Not only in New York, but all over the country, the doctors evinced a sudden enthusiasm respecting the Adirondacks that was obviously kindled by Dr. Loomis's torch. Limited as is the writer's own circle of acquaintance, he has been besieged in his wilderness retreat by letters of inquiry from those seeking the facts this volume is designed to furnish. Among other things wanted was Dr. Loomis's paper. Appearing as it did in a strictly technical journal, it could not, of course, reach the mass of unprofessional readers. That is why it has been thought well to include it in this book.

The writer hastens to add that the distinguished medical professor is not only not responsible for this republication of his essay, but he is ignorant even of its appropriation. Furthermore, the writer does not enjoy a personal acquaintance with Dr. Loomis. If he did, this public apology might not be called for. As it is, he sincerely hopes that the use of this material will not seem a misappropriation.

The article is given entire. All attempts to condense or abbreviate a purely technical article, written by a physician, are usually worse than vain. They are apt to do the medical author a positive injury. This was abundantly proved in the only newspaper extract of Dr. Loomis's paper which the writer has seen. Apart from that, although designed for professional ears, there is not a word in Dr. Loomis's report which will not be read with keen interest by every sufferer from phthisical disease.

DR. LOOMIS'S ADDRESS.

Mr. President and Gentlemen of the State Medical Society :—I invite your attention to the Adirondack region as a therapeutical agent in the treatment of pulmonary phthisis. I have long been convinced that the most important factor in the successful management of pulmonary phthisis is to be found in climate. It seems to me that at the present time no subject of medical study is more deserving of attention than the climatic treatment of disease, yet to a student of the medical literature of to-day there is none more confusing and unsatisfactory. Some localities have been considered especially favorable on account of their equability of temperature, others on account of

5

their luxurious vegetation or their peculiarity of soil; some on account of the dryness, others on account of the humidity of the atmosphere. From the data given, widely differing conclusions have been reached by different observers. In regard to the localities which are claimed to be especially adapted to the treatment of pulmonary phthisis, few writers have carefully observed, for any considerable length of time, the effect of the climate upon individual cases, or, if they have so observed, they have not made public the result of such observations; and on this account very definite conclusions as to the relative merits of the different localities have never been reached.

In the preparation of this paper, my object has been to show the effect of the climate of the Adirondack region upon all the cases of well-developed phthisis which, under my observation, have given the region an extended trial. I am largely indebted for facts given, and the history of cases, to my friend Dr. Edward L. Trudeau, who, with a phthisical invalid, took up his residence in this region five years ago.

By way of explanation, I would state that clinically and pathologically I recognize three varieties of pulmonary phthisis, viz., catarrhal phthisis, fibrous phthisis, and tubercular phthisis.

In *catarrhal phthisis*, the primary changes are in the cavities of the alveoli and bronchi, and are epithelial and cellular in their nature.

In *fibrous phthisis*, the primary changes occur in the bronchial and alveolar connective-tissue, and are connective-tissue hyperplasias.

In *tubercular phthisis*, the primary changes occur
in the lymphoid elements of the lung, associated with
connective-tissue hyperplasias forming little masses
or nodules, which ordinarily are termed tubercles.
The development of tubercle in a lung may be preceded or accompanied by an alveolar cellular process,
or by a connective-tissue hyperplasia, and as the one
or the other predominates, so is the duration of the
case long or short.

In the later stages of these different varieties of
phthisis, it is always difficult, and sometimes impossible, to distinguish the one from the other; but in
the earlier stages, in most cases, the differential diagnosis can readily be made.

The peculiar clinical feature of catarrhal phthisis
is, that at the onset the local symptoms are well
marked and precede or accompany the constitutional.·
The local signs may be those of pneumonia or of
localized bronchitis of the small tubes, while the
peculiar clinical feature of tubercular phthisis is, that
at the onset of the disease there are few local signs,
while the constitutional disturbance is very marked.

Fibrous phthisis is distinguished from all other
forms by its greater chronicity. Usually it commences
as a chronic affection, coming on very insidiously.
Its chief clinical feature is, that its development is
preceded by a chronic bronchitis or pleurisy limited
to one lung, or perhaps an unresolved pneumonia.
In rare instances, it is developed in the course of some
constitutional disease—as syphilis, gout, etc.

These three varieties of pulmonary phthisis not

only differ in their origin, mode of development, progress and termination, but necessarily they require different plans of treatment, and are differently affected by climate.

To rightly estimate the effect of the climate of any place or region, it is absolutely necessary that we be able to determine what variety of phthisis it is that is cured or arrested in that locality. Frequently, individuals with catarrhal phthisis will do badly at an altitude at which those with fibrous phthisis will be benefited. Besides, in determining the locality in which phthisical developments will be most likely to be arrested, we must take into account the age and general condition of the individual. For instance, an enfeebled and broken down middle-aged phthisical subject does badly in a high mountain region, but is benefited by the air of the sea.

The region known as the Adirondack region is comprised in that portion of our State which lies north of the Mohawk and west of the Champlain Valley. It may be said to include the counties of Clinton, Franklin, Essex, Hamilton, with portions of adjoining counties, and has an area equal in extent to nearly one-third of the State of New York. Within its limits there is a plateau from 1,500 to 2,000 feet above sea level, 150 miles in length (latitude), and 100 miles in breadth (longitude). On this plateau there are more than two thousand square miles of primitive forests, mostly evergreen, and many hundred lakes and ponds. From the surface of this plateau rise granitic mountain peaks more than five

thousand feet in height. The drainage of this table-
land is toward Lake Champlain on the east, the St.
Lawrence River on the northwest, and the Hudson
River on the south. Many of the streams which
flow in these different directions intercept each other,
and some of them, as well as the lakes, are navigable
for light canoes or boats. Occasionally there are
easy portages between these bodies of water, and
sometimes we meet with rapids or falls. I doubt
whether any region in this country furnishes to the
invalid or pleasure-seeker such a stimulus to out-of-
door life.

Mr. Verplanck Colvin, in the conclusion to his report, published in 1874, on the Topographical Survey
of the Adirondack Wilderness, uses the following
words to express his enthusiasm—words which fitly
express the enthusiasm of many another one familiar
with this region:

"The Adirondack wilderness may be considered
the wonder and glory of New York. It is a vast
natural park, one immense and silent forest, curi-
ously and beautifully broken by the gleaming waters
of a myriad of lakes, between which rugged mountain ranges rise as a sea of granite billows. At the
northeast the mountains culminate within an area of
some hundreds of square miles; and here savage,
treeless peaks, towering above the timber line, crowd
one another, and, standing gloomily shoulder to
shoulder rear their rocky crests amid the frosty
clouds. The wild beasts may look forth from the
ledges on the mountain sides over unbroken wood-

lands stretching beyond the reach of sight—beyond the blue hazy ridges at the horizon. The voyager by canoe beholds lakes in which these mountains and wild forests are reflected like inverted reality ; now wondrous in their dark grandeur and solemnity ; now glorious in resplendent autumn color of pearly beauty."

These words are the enthusiastic outbursts of one who has a more accurate and comprehensive knowledge of the topography of this region than has any other man.

It is not surprising that in such a region the tired worker and worn-out invalid find the rest and quiet which is so powerful a restorer of health. Here, as I have already intimated, there is every inducement for one to lead an out-of-door life ; the very surroundings infuse new life into the feeble body, and one daily grows stronger and stronger and feels better, scarcely able to tell how or why. One condition which I regard of the greatest importance in seeking a suitable home for the phthisical invalid is here met with, viz. : dryness of soil.

Undoubtedly a damp warm, as well as a damp cold, climate acts unfavorably upon phthisical invalids, but the peculiar *dampness* which acts most unfavorably is not usually present in those localities where there is the greatest rainfall, nor is it present because large bodies of water are in close proximity, but it mainly depends upon the nature of the soil. To avoid this dampness, the soil should be porous and sandy—a loose soil of sufficient porosity to permit the rapid filtering of water from its surface, so that after a heavy rainfall the surface will soon become dry. All clay soil drains slowly and imperfectly, and the peculiar dampness arises which acts so unfavorably on phthisical invalids.   Laennec states, that the dampness arising from such a condition of soil is one of the most certain developing causes of phthisis, and he makes mention of a locality, having such a soil, in which the dampness was so constant and of such a character, that more than two-thirds of the resident population died of phthisis.   In determining the fitness of a locality as a residence for phthisical invalids, I have come to regard the external configuration and conformation of the soil as of greater importance than the amount of rainfall, or the relative moisture.

The climate of the Adirondack region may be considered a moist, cool climate.   The rainfall is above the average for other portions of the State, and may be roughly estimated at fifty-five inches. The spring is cool, and there is considerable rain until about the middle of June.   There is a dry period during the summer, when little rain falls, and the days become hot, while almost without an exception the nights are cool, often cold, and heavy dews fall. There is rarely at any time excessive heat, and during the warmest weather there are but few nights, even in August, when a blanket is not needed.   My friend Dr. Trudeau, who has remained here summer and winter for the past five years, makes the following statement: "That he has never found the mercury above 87° during the past six summers, and this high temperature was only maintained for a few hours during the afternoon. The air during the fall months, with the exception of one or two long rain-storms, is bracing and admirably suited to out-of-door life. During the winter the cold is almost uninterrupted, no thawing of any consequence taking place before the month of March. There is a preponderance of cloudy days and snow-storms. The mercury, during January and February, frequently for days at a time stands many degrees below zero. As the cold weather usually continues until the end of March, the thawing takes place quickly, and owing to the sieve-like nature of the soil the snow disappears very rapidly, consequently the change from winter to spring is soon accomplished.

There is no marked preponderance of clear days at any season; on the contrary, the sky, especially in winter, is constantly overcast. This cool, cloudy weather is a marked feature of this climate. The altitude varies with the different localities; but the immense plateau which forms the lake region of the Adirondacks is about eighteen hundred feet above sea-level. The soil is very light and sandy, with here and there rocks, but little or no clay.

There appears at first sight but little to induce one to consider this locality as favorable for persons affected with phthisis. Hitherto heat and cold and absence of moisture, or an equable temperature, have been regarded as necessary in order to favorable results in the treatment of phthisis; but it has been shown by trial that neither cold, nor heat, nor moisture, alone, are all-sufficient factors in guiding us to a right understanding of the most favorable atmospheric conditions for phthisical patients. In a written communication to me, Dr. Trudeau also says: " High mountains, the desert, and the open sea, have perhaps given so far the best results in the treatment of chronic chest disease; and yet all these differ widely except in one respect, namely, purity of atmosphere. It is neither hot nor cold air, damp nor dry air, but *pure* air which is necessary to diseased lungs. Many conditions render the atmosphere of these mountains perfectly pure. The elevation of this region, its sandy soil, the undulating nature of the country, which ensures perfect drainage; the absence of cultivation, even of dwellings—all these conditions preclude the presence of telluric or miasmatic poison, and we have a purity of atmosphere unknown in more settled districts. The forests of this region are almost unbroken, stretching over the valleys, covering the mountains often to their very summit, and extending in some directions for nearly a hundred miles, while innumerable lakes dot this elevated plateau and give moisture to the air. That the atmosphere of such a region, especially when set in motion, should, by its contact with myriads of tree-tops and pine sheaves, become heavily laden with ozone is a natural sequence. Whatever other properties this gas may hereafter be found to possess, we know that it is a powerful disinfectant and Nature's choice agent for counteracting atmospheric impurities. This process, which during the summer months is carried on

5*

by all varieties of trees, during the winter months is
maintained by the evergreens, while the deciduous
trees are deprived of their foliage.   Pine, balsam,
spruce, and hemlock trees abound, and the air is
heavily laden with the resinous odors which they ex-
hale.   An agent which it is universally admitted ex-
erts a most beneficial influence on diseased mucous
membranes is thus brought in contact with the air-
passages, while balsamics, which are also disinfect-
ants, purify the atmosphere, which is constantly im-
pregnated with them.   Besides this, the air of the
wilderness is optically pure, noticeably free from dust
or visible particles of any kind.   The invalid, therefore, is here surrounded by a zone of pure air, which
separates him, as it were, from the germ-pervaded
world, and his diseased lungs are supplied with a
specially vitalized and purified atmosphere, free from
germs and impurities of any kind, and laden with
the resinous exhalations of myriads of evergreens."

Though as yet but few phthisical invalids have
been induced to give the Adirondack region an extended trial, the good results obtained by those who
have remained there for any considerable length of
time are the strongest arguments in its favor.   Dr.
Trudeau writes: "My own personal experience and
my personal observation of other phthisical invalids
lead me to say that any comparison of the relative
good effects of the climate of St. Paul, Minn., or of the
South, with that of the Adirondack region, is decidedly in favor of the latter."   In regard to camp life,
he writes: "Camping out, which is the peculiar fea-

ture of this place, if done in an intelligent manner, from June to October, I consider an important and beneficial measure in the treatment of phthisis; if done carelessly, it is by no means free from risk. The advantages gained by this mode of life are evident. The phthisical invalid for four months, night and day, lives out-of-doors, in a pure atmosphere; he is quiet, has perfect rest, plenty of good food (for which this mode of life gives an amazing relish); he has no opportunity to daily observe the effect upon other phthisical invalids of the disease from which he is suffering; his surroundings are such that he can lie down whenever standing fatigues him, can eat whenever he is hungry, sleep when exhausted, and dress as suits his own comfort—all of which comforts the requirements of society sometimes interfere with.

"All these things—the breathing of the pure air of the wilderness, the perfect rest, the wholesome food, and early hours—combine to make tent-life a powerful weapon in combating this disease.

"Exposure in inclement weather, which this mode of life at times renders almost unavoidable, is well borne in this climate by phthisical invalids who steadily live out of doors. During the past six years I have never seen any evil results from this mode of life; but I have seen men in camp lose their cough and gain in flesh while it rained daily, and in the midst of occasional frosts and snow-storms."

Dr. Trudeau expresses himself strongly on this point, having faithfully tried tent-life, and he adds: "Many of the risks supposed to attend out-of-door life exist only in the imagination of the timid ; " and he believes that tent-life, and a return to the invigorating, out-of-door existence of the savage is Nature's antidote for a disease which is almost an outgrowth of civilization and its enervating influences.

To proceed to results obtained from a fair trial of this region.

CASE I.—Eleven years ago, in the summer of 1867, as an invalid, I first visited this region. For several months previous I had suffered from cough with muco-purulent expectoration, loss of flesh and strength, night-sweats, and other rational and physical signs which attend incipient phthisical development. The only survivor of a family, every member of which (save, perhaps, one) had died of phthisis, I had come to regard my case a critical one. A Southern trip had not relieved, if it had not aggravated, my phthisical symptoms. In this condition I went into this region and into camp, and when, before the summer months had passed, I came out of the Adirondack or north woods free from cough, with an increase in weight of about twenty pounds, with greater physical vigor than I had known for years, I very naturally became an enthusiast in regard to them.

My personal experience that summer convinced me that there was something in the air of this region especially adapted to diseased lungs ; that, if the climate had no direct influence in arresting or preventing phthisical developments, it certainly allayed bronchial irritation, and the phthisical invalid soon became able to spend the greater portion of his time

in the open air ; still more, his surroundings were
such that if a lover of nature or of sport, he necessarily forgot himself, and thus was nature aided, and
vigor and health restored.

I would mention here that my personal experience,
as well as my experience since that time in regard to
its effect upon others, leads me to believe that, during the warm season, a camp or tent-life is of the
greatest service to pulmonary invalids, if they are
not enfeebled.

From time to time, since that summer, eleven
years ago, I have sent phthisical invalids into this
region. At first I sent them only during the summer months, but I found that while temporary relief
was afforded, and in some instances marked improvement took place, in cases of fully developed phthisis
the latter was not permanent, and although the winter months might be spent at the South, yet before
another summer came around the disease progressed.
Not until 1873 was I able to persuade any phthisical
invalid to remain during the winter. The effect of
the winter climate on this invalid showed so markedly the benefit to be derived from a winter's residence
in this region, that from that time, each winter,
others have been induced to remain. Fourteen remained last winter.

A brief analysis of the cases which have been
under my own personal supervision, or that of Dr.
Trudeau, will, I think, enable us to reach some satisfactory conclusions in regard to the therapeutical
effects of the climate of the Adirondack region. They

are unselected cases, and the only cases of value, as these are the only phthisical invalids who have remained in the region a sufficient length of time to give the climate anything like a fair trial.

CASE II.—Dr. E. L. T——, aged twenty-five; family history good; began to lose his health in the winter of 1872. His symptoms were rapidly becoming urgent; he was examined by several physicians. Extensive consolidation at left apex was found, extending posteriorly nearly to angle of scapula; on the right side nothing was discovered save slight pleuritic adhesions at the apex.

He was ordered South, but returned in the spring in no way benefited. On the contrary, night-sweating had set in, and his fever was higher. In the latter part of May he started for the Adirondacks, the ride in the stage being accomplished on an improvised bed. His condition at this time was most unpromising; he had daily fever, night-sweats, profuse and purulent expectoration, had lost his appetite, and was obliged constantly to have recourse to stimulants. Weight about one hundred and thirty-four pounds. He began to improve at once, his appetite returned, all his symptoms decreased in severity, and after a stay of more than three months he returned to New York, weighing one hundred and forty-six pounds, with only slight morning cough, presenting the appearance of a man in good health. A few days after his arrival in New York he had a chill, all his old symptoms returned, and he was advised to leave for St. Paul, where he spent the entire winter. He did badly there; was sick the greater portion of the winter. In the spring of 1873 he again went to the Adirondacks. At this time he was in a most debilitated state, was anæmic, emaciated, had daily hectic fever, constant cough, and profuse purulent expectoration.

The marked improvement did not commence at once, as it did the previous summer, and the first of September found him in a wretched condition. I then examined him for the first time, and found complete consolidation of the left lung over the scapula and supra-scapula space, with pleuritic thickenings and adhesions over the infra-clavicular space. On coughing, bronchial râles of large and small size were heard over the consolidated portion of the lung. Over the right infra-clavicular region the respiratory murmur was feeble, and on full inspiration pleuritic friction sounds were heard. I advised him to remain at St. Regis Lake during the winter, and although he was repeatedly warned that such a step would prove fatal, he followed my advice.

From that time he began slowly to improve. Since that time he has lived in this region. At the present time his weight is one hundred and fifty-eight pounds, a gain of twenty-two pounds since he first went to the Adirondacks in 1873, and ten pounds more than was his weight in health. He has slight morning cough and expectoration, his pulse is from 72 to 85, and he presents the appearance of a person in good health. In his lungs evidences still remain of the disease he has so many years combated.

Although he has made three attempts to live in New York, at intervals of two years, each time his removal from the mountains has been followed within ten days by a chill, and a return of pneumonic symptoms—symptoms so ominous that he has become convinced that it will be necessary for him to remain in the Adirondack region for some time to come.

CASE III.—In the fall of 1873, Mr. E——, aged twenty, with decided hereditary tendency to phthisis, went into the lake region of the Adirondacks. He had then been ill about eighteen months, had spent two winters in Nassau, and for the three months immediately preceding his arrival, he had failed very rapidly. When he first consulted me, in September, 1873, I found him extremely emaciated, weighing one hundred and eight pounds, pulse habitually ranging from 110 to 130, morning temperature from 102° to 103°. He had loss of appetite, night-sweats, and a constant harassing cough with slight hemorrhages. Physical examination revealed a large cavity on the right side posteriorly, with entire consolidation of the right lung. At the left apex there was also a small cavity with fine crackling râles over the upper third of the left lung. His condition remained desperate during the following winter, but in the spring he somewhat recovered his appetite, he regained strength, and he had long intervals during which he was entirely free from fever. He spent the spring and summer of 1874 in camp, and his improvement was very marked. A physical examination of his chest in the fall of 1874 showed a marked decrease in the pulmonary consolidation on the right side, the cavity had apparently diminished in size, and vesicular murmurs could be heard below and on either side of it.   On the left side the crackling sounds had disappeared, and no signs of cavity could longer be detected, but broncho-vesicular breathing was still distinctly heard.   His heart was hypertrophied, pulse 88, evening tempera-ture $99\frac{1}{4}°$, weight one hundred and sixteen pounds. For the succeeding eight months he steadily improved. In June, 1875, after an exposure which it would have been unwise for one in health to risk, he was seized with a prolonged chill, which was very severe, and was followed by a pulmonary hemorrhage so profuse that for some time he was thought to be dead, but he lingered until morning, and died from pulmonary con-gestion and œdema.

Although this case terminated fatally, I regarded it as one of arrested phthisis.   The beneficial effects of the climate of this lake region were so positive and well-marked in this case, that I assumed the responsi-bility and induced other phthisical invalids to make a trial of it, contrary to the advice of other physicians, and regardless of the expostulations of friends.

CASE IV.—Mr. M——, aged twenty-seven, with a good family history, after an illness of several months, which was marked by cough, expectoration, and loss of flesh, spent the summer of 1870 at Saranac Lake, where he markedly improved, lost his cough, and gained in weight.   After his return to New York in the fall, his cough returned, other physical symptoms developed, and he was quite ill throughout the winter. The next summer he returned to the Adirondacks much worse than he was the previous year. Again he improved, and he thought he was almost well. He went to California for the winter, did badly there, and on his return to New York in the spring, two physicians of large experience pronounced his case a hopeless one—one which would probably terminate fatally within six months. In the early summer of 1872 he reached the Adirondacks in a most pitiable condition. Both lungs were extensively diseased. At the apex of the left lung were the physical signs of extensive consolidation and softening. The upper third of the right lung was consolidated, and was the seat of large and small mucous râles. He had hectic fever, extreme dyspnœa, a rapid pulse, and other symptoms of advanced phthisis. He soon began to gain flesh and strength, his appetite improved, he coughed less, his expectoration was diminished in quantity, and by early fall he was able to keep out of doors the greater portion of the time. For five years he remained in the lake region. At times his condition was most promising, although little change took place in the physical signs. Last spring, tired of the seclusion, he returned to his home in New York.

Unquestionably this was a case of catarrhal phthisis, and the results obtained from his first summer's residence in the Adirondack region lead me to believe that if Mr. M. had remained in the region the winter succeeding this first summer, he would have reached complete recovery. Even after reaching an advanced stage of the disease, when there was no longer a possibility of recovery, a condition of stasis was reached when he permanently resided in the region.

CASE V.—Mrs. L——, aged forty, good family history; early in the summer of 1871 went to the Adirondacks. She had been ill eight months with a cough and other phthisical symptoms. At the time of her arrival she was in a state of extreme exhaustion; for several weeks previous she had lived entirely upon beef-tea and champagne. She had a harassing cough, with profuse expectoration, and hectic fever. Physical examination revealed a moderate amount of consolidation at the apex of the right lung, with crackling râles of large and small size; no evidence of softening. At once her desire for food returned, and she began to gain flesh and strength; gradually her cough and expectoration diminished, and late in the fall she returned to her home markedly improved. Since that time she has spent some time every summer or fall in this region, and for the last three years none of the rational or physical signs of phthisis have been present.

In this case the rapidity and completeness of the recovery was quite surprising, when we consider how unpromising was the condition of the patient at the time when she first reached the Adirondacks.

CASE VI.—Mr. R——, aged thirty, with no hereditary tendency to any disease, first consulted me in the spring of 1875. He had been ill six months with cough, expectoration, hectic fever, gradual emaciation, and other well-marked phthisical symptoms. Physical examination of chest revealed consolidation

at the apex of the right lung, with sharp crackling
râles, most abundant posteriorly, where distinct bronchial breathing could be heard below the spine of
the scapula; left lung healthy. I advised him to
take up his residence in the Adirondacks. He remained in camp in the lake region during the summer of 1875, with only a slight increase in weight, a
slight improvement in strength, and no change in
cough or physical signs. During the fall and winter
he had several hemorrhages, with fever, and was confined to his bed at different times. Early the next
spring he went into camp, and remained until September. When he came out of camp he weighed
one hundred and eighty-one pounds, had gained
forty pounds; he had no cough, no expectoration, no
fever. An examination of his chest revealed no abnormal sound, except pleuritic creaking and feeble
respiratory murmur posteriorly over the former seat
of the pulmonary consolidation. I regarded him a
well man, and permitted him to return to his home.
He remained well until the following spring, when
he had an attack of acute cystitis. He was confined
to his bed for six weeks; as soon as he was able to
travel he returned to the Adirondacks, but the cystitis became chronic, was complicated by pyélitis and
nephritis, and in early winter he died from acute
uræmia.

At the time Mr. R. took up his residence in the
Adirondacks, his digestive and assimilating processes
were in a feeble condition. Undoubtedly this ac-
counted for the fact that for nearly a year there was

little, if any, improvement in his lung disease. His five months' camp life during the second year of his residence in the Adirondacks not only cured his diseased lung, but wrought an entire change in his physical condition. So great was the change, that one would scarcely recognize him. When he left the woods the following fall, no evidence of lung disease could be detected, nor was any detected during the remainder of his life.

CASE VII.—Miss C——, aged eighteen, in the spring or early summer of 1875 reached the Adirondacks in a very feeble condition. She had had a cough for six months, with frequent pulmonary hemorrhages, attended by fever, loss of flesh and strength. Physical examination of the chest revealed dulness on percussion, bronchial respiration, and crackling râles at the apex of the right lung. Her improvement began at once; at the expiration of three months she had gained eleven pounds in weight, had no cough, and had so regained her strength as to be able to take active out-of-door exercise. In early fall she returned to her home, and has there remained in good health.

In this case the pulmonary consolidation was evidently catarrhal in its nature, and of recent date. That she came to the Adirondacks in the earlier stages of the disease, probably had much to do with her rapid and complete recovery.

CASE VIII.—Mr. B——, aged thirty-two, with a decided hereditary predisposition to phthisis, took up his residence in the lake region of the Adirondacks

in the summer of 1875. After he left home, before
he reached the Adirondacks, he had a severe hemorrhage. For three months after his arrival he was
in a critical condition, had severe cough, frequent
hemorrhages, fever, and rapid emaciation. He did
not begin to improve until late in the fall, after
which time his improvement was steadily progressive.
During a two years' residence in the region he fully
regained health and strength, his cough ceased, and
in August, 1878, I could find no trace of disease in
the lungs, except old pleuritic thickenings and adhesions at the apex of the left lung. In September,
1878, he left the Adirondacks.

During his first year's residence in the Adirondacks
no physical examination was made, but he stated that
previous to his coming into the region his medical
advisers had told him that his lungs were extensively
diseased, and that he had come with a "forlorn
hope." His disease commenced as a "severe cold,"
and unquestionably his case was one of catarrhal
phthisis.

CASE IX—Dr. T——, aged thirty-two, with marked
hereditary tendency to phthisis, came to the Adirondacks in the summer of 1875. For ten months he
had been ill with well-marked phthisical symptoms.
The upper third of the right lung was consolidated,
with circumscribed liquid râles in the supra-scapular
fossa. At the apex of the left lung there was exaggerated rude respiration, but no râles. He remained
four months, in camp the greater portion of the
time. As he improved he became restless, and could

not be induced to longer remain. His weight was now one hundred and forty-eight pounds, he had gained twelve pounds, and had no cough. After leaving the Adirondacks he went South, but returned in the spring in a most enfeebled condition; weight one hundred and twenty-seven pounds, with pallid countenance, difficult breathing, and so weak that he was obliged to lie down the greater portion of the time. The entire upper lobe of the lung on the right side was consolidated, and abundant râles were heard throughout the consolidated portion. The respirations at the apex of the left lung had become markedly bronchial in character. He began to improve, and by the first of December had regained his appetite and strength. Again he became restless, left the Adirondacks, went to Colorado and California, was twice near death, and in early summer returned to the Adirondacks "in extremis," with a large cavity in his right lung, and commencing softening in his left lung. Having thrown away his chances for recovery, he died in early winter.

A series of mistakes marked the course of this patient. A short time previous to his death he stated to me that in attempting to follow the advice of his Philadelphia physician, who recommended a warm climate, and that of his New York medical adviser, who recommended a cold climate, he had made the result a failure.

As we review his history, it seems to me that we are warranted in coming to the conclusion that the result might have been different had he remained in

the Adirondack region for two or three years succeeding his first visit.

CASE X.—Mrs. M——, aged twenty-eight, with no
hereditary tendency to phthisis, consulted me in the
fall of 1876. She had a cough, which was paroxysmal
in character, with little expectoration. For several
months she had been losing flesh, had had daily
fever and night-sweats; at times she had suffered
from severe attacks of dyspnœa, which were followed
by an expectoration which she termed "stringy."
Physical examination revealed pulmonary consolidation posteriorly at the apex of the right lung, with
sharp bronchial râles over the consolidation. At different points over the chest, dry and moist râles were
heard, and I made the diagnosis of probable fibrous
bronchitis, with pulmonary consolidation at the apex
of the right lung. I advised her to spend the winter
in Asheville, N. C., where she obtained little, if any,
relief. During the winter she expectorated a number of well-formed bronchial casts. On her return, I
found her more feeble than when I first saw her, and
the area of lung consolidation increased.

Following my advice, in June she went into the
lake region of the Adirondacks, remained nearly a
year, and entirely recovered from the bronchitis and
pulmonary consolidation.

This case was one of well-marked plastic bronchitis, with circumscribed consolidation at the apex of
the right lung. When we recall the fact that the
majority of cases of chronic plastic bronchitis are
followed by phthisis, and terminate fatally, the com-

plete recovery reached in this case is somewhat surprising.

I would call attention to the fact that in this case the climate of the Adirondacks produced such different results from that of Asheville, N. C.

CASE XI.—Miss F——, aged nineteen, of a nonphthisical family, consulted me in March, 1875, having taken cold the previous January. She was rapidly losing flesh, had an almost constant hacking cough, night-sweats, with other well-marked phthisical symptoms. On physical examination, I found complete consolidation of the upper third of the right lung, with crackling râles posteriorly. Evening temperature 103°, and pulse feeble. She had lost ten pounds since January, and was easily exhausted. Ten days after I first saw her she had a profuse hemorrhage; in two days this was followed by a second. She was so reduced in strength by these hemorrhages, and her general symptoms became so aggravated, that unless soon arrested it was evident her pulmonary disease would progress very rapidly, and soon terminate fatally; I feared acute phthisis.

In the early part of April she went to Washington, was carried to and from the cars; she remained six weeks, with very little improvement in her condition, the entire upper lobe of the right lung having now become involved in the pulmonary consolidation. The early part of July she reached the Adirondacks. She rapidly began to improve, and when I examined her the following October, she had gained twenty pounds in weight, coughed only in the morning after

6

rising, had no fever, and had a pulse of 80. Bronchial breathing was heard posteriorly over the area of the pulmonary consolidation, while quite extensive pleuritic adhesions and thickening could be detected in front. She spent portions of the summer and fall months in the Adirondacks for the two succeeding years, and now regards herself perfectly well, and is so regarded by her friends.

The pleuritic changes which occurred during the active progress of the disease alone give evidence of her former pulmonary disease. When this patient first went to the Adirondacks, not only did her disease involve a large amount of lung-tissue, but her general condition was very unpromising, her stomach was exceedingly irritable, and her emaciation was rapid and her anæmia extreme.

CASE XII.—Mrs. P——, aged forty, from a non-phthisical family, first came under my observation in March, 1877. Since 1869 she had suffered with phthisical symptoms; at times her case had been regarded as hopeless. Physical examination revealed fibrous induration of the upper lobe of the right lung, with the physical signs of cavity under the right clavicle, and pleuritic thickening over the entire lung. Pulse 100, feeble, and easily accelerated. Temperature 101°; extreme dyspnœa consequent upon exertion. She had night-sweats, was extremely anæmic, not markedly emaciated, but her weight was less than when in health. Cough paroxysmal and violent, with slate-colored expectoration; her appetite was capricious, and her disease had made marked progress since

the early part of January.   In early summer she went
to the lake region, where she remained until fall.   In
her general health the improvement was very marked ;
but little change took place in the physical signs.
During the winter there was little change in her condition.   Early the following summer (summer of
1878) she went to the Adirondacks and into camp,
where she remained until the following October.
Not only was the improvement in her general health
very marked, but her cough almost entirely disappeared, and her general physical condition was better
than it had been since the commencement of her disease.   The fibrous induration remained at the apex
of the right lung, although vesicular breathing could
be heard over the remaining portion of the lung.

When I first examined this case I regarded it as
one of fibrous phthisis, and only hoped for that complete cicatricial process to be developed which renders
the diseased lung-tissue inactive.   While, as yet, she
has not reached such a condition, her steady improvement without any new lung-tissue becoming involved,
and the absence of any evidence that degenerative
processes have been developed in the lung-tissue
already involved, leads me to believe that if the same
climatic influences be continued, which during the
past two years have produced such beneficial results,
at length the desired result may be obtained.

CASE XIII.—Mr. S——, aged thirty-one, with a
good family history ; at my suggestion went to the
Adirondacks in the early part of the summer of 1876.

He first consulted me in the fall of 1875, had then

been ill about one year; had well-marked phthisical symptoms. He had received a most unfavorable prognosis from medical men in this country and in Europe. A physical examination revealed quite extensive consolidation of the apex of the right lung, with sharp crackling râles. I advised him to spend the winter in Asheville, N. C. On his return in early summer, I found that although his general condition had somewhat improved, his pulmonary disease had made considerable progress. Soon after his arrival in the Adirondacks he was seized with an acute cystitis, which prostrated him very much. Although he remained nearly two years in the lake region, his pulmonary disease steadily, but slowly, progressed. In the spring of 1878, in an extremely debilitated condition, he returned to his home in Ohio.

In this case, the disease from its onset steadily progressed, and the diagnosis of tubercular phthisis which was made the first time I saw him, was confirmed by his subsequent history. While he was in the Adirondack region, although at times he seemed to be improving, the periods of improvement were of short duration, and each exacerbation of fever left him in a more and more enfeebled condition. With each exacerbation of fever, new areas of lung-tissue became involved. At the time he left for his home in Ohio, suspicious bubbling sounds were heard over the original seat of his disease, and his respirations were amphoric in character.

CASE XIV.—Mr. L——, aged twenty-two, with well-marked phthisical symptoms, had been ill six

months, when, in the summer of 1877, he took up
his residence in the Adirondacks.   At the time of
his arrival his cough was constant, his expectoration
was of a greenish color, and of tenacious consistency.
He was rapidly losing flesh, had night-sweats, and
shortness of breath upon slight exertion.   Physical
examination revealed consolidation at the apex of the
right lung, with fine crackling râles in the supra-scapular fossa.   He remained about one year, spending
the summer and early fall in camp.   His cough disappeared, and he gained fourteen pounds in weight.
Ten months after his arrival no abnormal sound could
be heard in his lungs, except feeble respiratory murmur, and pleuritic creaking at the end of a full inspiration at the former seat of the pulmonary consolidation.   He has continued perfectly well to the
present time, and is now studying law.   This was a
case of catarrhal phthisis in its first stage, in which,
like the previous case of which I have made mention, the recovery from the pulmonary disease was
rapid and complete.

CASE XV.—Mrs. G——, of a non-phthisical family, first consulted me in April, 1878.   She had suffered with well-marked phthisical symptoms for six
months, the result of a cold contracted the previous
summer, while she was in a debilitated condition,
which had been followed by a cough.   Physical examination of the chest revealed consolidation of the
upper two-thirds of the right lung, with circumscribed
moist râles under the right clavicle with amphoric
breathing.   She was very feeble; had rapidly lost

flesh; had night-sweats, loss of appetite, an almost constant cough, an abundant expectoration, with occasional spitting of blood, and dyspnœa upon slight exertion. Temperature in the evening, 103°; pulse, 110 to 120.

She went into the lake region of the Adirondacks in June, and returned the last of September. She made little or no improvement until the last of August; from that time she began to rapidly improve, and has continued to gain flesh to the present time. She now weighs thirty-eight pounds more than before she went to the Adirondacks, and coughs only in the morning. Physical examination shows vesicular breathing over the seat of the former consolidation, except posteriorly, where the breathing is broncho-vesicular in character, and pleuritic creakings are well marked. No signs of cavity can be detected.

The improvement in this case did not commence until two months after she reached the Adirondacks; in fact, for a time the disease seemed to be progressing with some degree of rapidity. During this time she had two quite profuse hemorrhages. The changes in the diseased lung were so extensive, and of such a nature, that I did not hope for recovery. The increase in weight has been greater and more rapid than in any other case of phthisis which has come under my observation.

CASE XVI.—Mr. R——, aged thirty, of a phthisical family, began to cough in the winter of 1876. Two months after he began to cough he had a hemorrhage. Soon after the hemorrhage he began to have fever and to lose flesh. He first consulted me in May, 1876. He then presented the appearance of one in advanced phthisis. He was emaciated, had an evening temperature of 102° and 103°, and had great difficulty of breathing, becoming exhausted from the exertion attending the ascent of a flight of stairs. Physical examination revealed extensive consolidation of the upper lobe of the right lung. Distinct bronchial respiration could be heard from the clavicle to the upper border of the fourth rib. He went into the Adirondack region, where he remained a year. On his return to New York he presented the appearance of perfect health. He had no cough, and said he weighed more, and felt stronger and better than he had for years. Physical examination revealed only pleuritic thickening over the former seat of the pulmonary consolidation. No physical examination of the chest was made from the time he went into the Adirondack region in early winter until his return to New York, one year later. He stated that his improvement commenced about three weeks after he reached the Adirondacks, and that every day during the winter months he spent from six to eight hours out of doors.

He has remained in New York until the present time, and has had no return of his phthisical symptoms.

Case XVII.—Mr. A——, aged thirty-one, with a strong hereditary tendency to phthisis, had his first hemorrhage in February, 1877, after which he rapidly lost flesh and strength, and in June, when I first saw him, he was extremely emaciated and anæmic; had a constant hacking cough, with muco-purulent expectoration, and frequent slight hemorrhages. Temperature ranged from 100° to 103°; pulse never below 100, and easily accelerated. Physical examination revealed slight consolidation at both apices, with moist, bubbling râles in left supra-scapular fossa. He went into the Adirondacks in July, and remained nearly a year, during which time his disease slowly, but steadily, progressed. A physical examination in July, 1878, revealed a cavity at the apex of the left lung, with infiltration of the entire left lung. I advised his return to his family.

In this case the diagnosis of tubercular phthisis· was made at the first examination. The subsequent history and the uninterrupted progress of the disease fully sustained the diagnosis first made.

CASE XVIII.—Mrs. O——, aged thirty-four, with no hereditary predisposition to phthisis, first consulted me in May, 1878. She had coughed for six months, had repeatedly had hemorrhages. She went South during the winter of 1877–78, where she did badly, rapidly losing health and strength, and had afternoon fever and night-sweats. Pulse 102° F., feeble and easily accelerated. Afternoon temperature 102°. She complained of dyspnœa on slight exertion, and became easily fatigued, was anæmic, had no desire for food, and was dyspeptic. A physical examination revealed consolidation of the upper third of the left lung, with bronchial râles and pleuritic adhesions over the entire left side.

In July she went to St. Regis Lake (Adirondacks), where she remained three months. Immediately she began to improve; the cough became less and less troublesome, her appetite returned, and she soon gained fourteen pounds in weight. By the first of September her pulse and temperature were normal, and by the first of October the only physical evidences of disease were slight pulmonary consolidation under left scapula, and pleuritic creaking in left infra-clavicular space. She has continued to improve since her return, and is now apparently well.

This was another case in which the rapid and continued improvement was unexpected. The general appearance and condition of the patient when first seen by me was unpromising. The perseverance or fixedness of purpose, and good sense of the patient, I believe had very much to do with her marked improvement. She remained out of doors nearly the whole of every day, took no risks, and made use of everything in her surroundings which would aid in bringing about the desired result.

CASE XIX.—Mr. M——, aged thirty-four, consulted me in the spring of 1877, having had a pulmonary hemorrhage. For the previous three months he had been rapidly losing flesh and strength, had fever, night-sweats, and was extremely anæmic. He had had cough with expectoration for more than a year. Physical examination revealed consolidation of the apex of the left lung as far as the lower border of the third rib, with quite extensive pleuritic changes and marked retraction of the left side of the

6*

chest. He had repeated hemorrhages, was confined to his room for several weeks, and it was the latter part of June before he was able to travel. Early in July he started for the Adirondacks. He presented the appearance of a person in advanced phthisis, and physical examination at this time detected marked retraction of the left chest and bronchial dilatation in the left supra-scapular space.

During July and August his improvement was very slight, and it was the latter part of August before he was able to go into camp. He remained about two months in camp, during which time he regained his normal weight, his strength returned, and he had great physical endurance. Late in the fall he returned to New York, presenting the appearance of one in health, although he still had cough and shortness of breath, and physical examination showed little change in the consolidated lung. His improvement continued until the following March, when he again grew worse, lost flesh, and had occasional fever. In May he had another slight hemorrhage. An examination of his chest showed an increase in the pulmonary consolidation since the previous examination; pleuritic adhesions and thickenings were detected over the whole of the left side, with more marked retraction on the left side. He again went to the Adirondacks, and remained in camp the greater portion of the summer and fall. He rapidly regained flesh and strength, and all his active phthisical symptoms again disappeared, excepting morning cough with expectoration. Little change could be detected in his physical signs. Unquestionably this is a case of fibrous phthisis, and although while he remains in the Adirondacks he regains his flesh and strength, and the progress of the disease seems to be arrested, yet little or no improvement can be detected in the diseased lung.

CASE XX.—Miss H—— had her first pulmonary hemorrhage, which was quite profuse, in January, 1877. Within the week following this first hemorrhage she had frequent hemorrhages, averaging more than one per day. During the preceding year her physical and mental labor had been unusually taxing or severe, and she was not in her usual health. For several months she had suffered more or less from nasal, pharyngeal, and bronchial catarrh. She first consulted me in June, 1877, at which time she presented all the symptoms of well-developed phthisis. She had constant cough, with muco-purulent expectoration frequently streaked with blood, was emaciated, had fever, night-sweats, loss of appetite, shortness of breath, etc.

A physical examination revealed consolidation of left lung from its apex down to the fourth rib, with abundant mucous râles over the left scapula. In the early part of July she went into the Adirondacks, and into camp. On her return from the region in November, I found her much improved ; she coughed little, had no fever, had gained eight pounds in weight, could walk long distances without fatigue or shortness of breath. Physical examination showed marked diminution in pulmonary consolidation in the left infra-clavicular space; bronchial respiration and mucous râles were still heard over left scapula. She steadily improved until the middle of February, when she had a severe attack of influenza, from the effects of which she did not entirely recover, and June, 1878, found her in a worse condition than she was in June, 1877. Following the influenza, a pleurisy was established over the whole of the left pleura. This greatly increased her difficulty of respiration. June 11th she again left for the Adirondacks, went into camp July 1st, and remained in camp until October 10th. During the summer she had two slight hemorrhages, but she steadily regained her strength and weight, and seldom coughed. A physical examination, made the following November, showed entire absence of pulmonary consolidation at the apex of the left lung, and the only remaining physical signs of disease were pleuritic adhesions or thickenings over the upper third of the lung, with localized bronchial râles in the left supra-scapular fossa. Since November her improvement has been steadily progressive; she has the appearance of one in health, yet she has slight cough with muco-purulent expectoration, and physical signs of disease are still present.

The statement previously made in regard to the probable effect of a longer stay in the woods, holds true in this case.

A brief summary of the foregoing cases gives the following results:

Of the twenty persons who have tested the therapeutical power of the climate of the Adirondack region, by giving it an extended trial, ten have recovered, six have been improved, two have not been benefited, and two have died.

The ten cases of recovery were those of catarrhal phthisis; of the six cases in which improvement took place, four were those of catarrhal phthisis, and two were cases of fibrous phthisis. The two cases in which no benefit was received from a stay in the region were cases of tubercular phthisis, in both of which the disease steadily progressed, and at no time could it be said that it was even temporarily arrested. In both cases of fibrous phthisis, extensive retraction of lung had taken place, with bronchial dilatation and compensatory emphysematous developments. Exercise could not be taken, for very slight physical exertion brought on attacks of severe and frequent dyspnœa, and the severe attacks of coughing interfered with digestion and nutrition. In both cases failure of the right heart was well marked. In both the improvement manifested itself in the gaining of flesh and strength, rather than in any change in the lungs which could be appreciated by physical examination. I believe these cases would have done better in Colorado.

Those cases of catarrhal phthisis which were improved, but not cured, were those in which the pulmonary changes were extensive, or had reached the stage of excavation—cases in which complete recovery is always problematical.

In all these cases the improvement did not commence immediately—not until some time after the individual had taken up his residence in the region; and when it did commence, it was not constantly progressive. Each case had a long history of getting better and worse, but each advance toward recovery was more marked than the former. Whether these cases will or will not reach complete recovery, is a question, but I am certain that a permanent residence in the region greatly increases the probabilities of such a result, from the fact that in those cases which have come under my observation a temporary absence from this region has been followed by such sad results. In all the cases of catarrhal phthisis which have reached recovery, either the pulmonary changes were not extensive, or they were of recent origin, and improvement commenced soon after reaching the Adirondacks. The results obtained established the fact, that a large proportion of the cases of this variety of phthisis, if they have not passed the first stage, or stage of consolidation, can recover.

The two cases that terminated fatally were cases of catarrhal phthisis. Although, when they came into this region, their lungs were extensively diseased, they were much benefited during their stay, and it seems to me that impatience and imprudence had very much to do with the fatal termination.

Results show that the climate of this region is better adapted to the treatment of catarrhal phthisis than of any other variety. I believe fibrous phthisis does better in higher altitudes—for instance, in Colorado.

My experience leads me to believe that climate has little beneficial effect upon tubercular phthisis.

For some time I have believed—in fact I became convinced soon after I began to study carefully the effect of climate upon phthisical invalids—that a larger proportion of such were benefited or cured in a cold than in a warm climate.

The testimony of those who have spent a winter, or more than one winter, in the Adirondacks is, that improvement was far more rapid during the winter than during the summer months; and I have found, by physical examination of the lungs, that the arrest in the morbid processes and the establishment of the curative processes was more marked during the winter than during the summer months.

I shall have accomplished my purpose, if by this hastily prepared paper I shall have awakened in my professional brethren the spirit of investigation as regards this extensive health-restoring region, within the boundaries of our own State, which we have been passing by, while we have sent phthisical invalids far from home and friends to regions far less restorative.

CHAPTER X.

THE COST OF THE THING.

In dealing with the matter of expense, as connected with the wilderness experiment, it has been thought advisable to put the information under a separate heading, instead of scattering it over the pages of this little volume.

The cost of any undertaking of this sort will, of course, depend largely on the tastes and circumstances of the invalid. To the fortunate few whom fate has in some measure compensated for the loss of health by bestowing large fortunes upon them, this chapter will be of little moment. They may omit it altogether in deciding upon the trip. To that infinitely larger number, however, who must consult their purses before carrying out any plan, even where that plan may involve the question of life or death, the money item assumes no insignificant proportions. And for those who are called upon to bear the burden of actual poverty with that of wasting disease—those who have heretofore looked upon a journey to the established health-resorts as among the bitter impossibilities which poverty imposes—for those it will be

a gracious duty to point the way to this new El
Dorado whose gold is life.

As a convenient starting-point in the calculations
which are to follow, we will suppose the health-seeker
to have reached the most important gateway of the
upper wilderness—Plattsburg. The fare from that
town to the St. Regis Lake House by the present
route is $4.50. Each passenger is allowed one trunk
by the stage, and will be charged an extra $2 for
each additional trunk. Dinner at the half-way house,
seventy-five cents.

The established price for board at "Paul" Smith's
is $2.50 per day. Unlike any other house of its
character of which the writer has any knowledge, no
deduction from the per-diem rates is made on account of a prolonged stay. The guest pays $2.50 if
he remains a day, and at precisely the same rate if
he remains four months.

Guides consider their services worth $2.50 per day
and their board. The hotel sets a separate table for
their accommodation, at which meals are served for
twenty-five cents each. When engaged in the work
of guiding proper, the men fairly earn all they get.
When employed regularly in the permanent camp
of an invalid, it must be confessed that $17.50 a
week, with board included, is a rate of wages for un-
skilled labor out of all keeping with existing values.
The men themselves understand this fact, and where
one can be found willing to attend an invalid, he
may generally be hired for $1 a day. In all such
cases it is understood that the place is to be permanent

for the season, provided, of course, the man proves satisfactory.

Where it is possible, it is best to hire a guide who owns a boat. Otherwise one may be rented from the hotel at fifty cents a day. When new, these boats cost from $40 to $75. A good second-hand one may often be bought in the autumn as low as $15.

A good canvas tent, ten by twelve feet, can be purchased in New York for about $35. This might not include poles and stakes, but as it costs much more than their value to transport these, they are better left behind. A covering or fly for the tent may be made of heavy cotton cloth, which serves the purpose quite as well as canvas.

For the ordinary labor required in preparing a permanent camp, $1 a day, with the man's board, is a fair allowance. A good strong woman for kitchen work ought to be found for $3 a week. Boys (if any can be found small enough or young enough not to regard themselves as guides) may be employed for fifty cents a day. No other kind of labor need be considered, as there are no regular mechanics or artisans in the region.

In the necessary furniture of a camp, a very small outlay will meet the requirements, if the items of stoves and beds be excepted. For the former, a good cook-stove may sometimes be hired from the year-round inhabitants, the user paying two or three dollars for the season. This is the most economical way. A tent-stove of sheet-iron costs, perhaps, $5, with something more for the pipe. A good bed is the most expensive necessity of the sick man's camp. The hotel furnishes blankets for roughing it, but it will not be well to depend on this source for a comfortable and civilized bed. Those who set out with an eye to economy cannot do better than bring their bed with them—that is, a good mattress, pillows and blankets, with enough of the last to meet the colder nights safely.

The staple articles of food are sold, as a rule, at a considerable advance on the New York market prices, but to this statement exception must be made in the matter of eggs, butter, and milk. The very best of butter was supplied us at fifteen to twenty cents per pound. The highest price for eggs was twenty cents per dozen. Rich, creamy milk could be had for five cents a quart. Spring lambs can be bought for from $2 to $3, which reduces the price of delicious chops, roasts, and stews, to something under ten cents per pound. Beef sells at the hotel for twenty cents a pound—but Adirondack beef would be dear at twenty pounds for a cent. Venison brings from ten to twelve cents a pound. Chickens are plentiful at twenty-five cents apiece. Trout, in their season, if sold at all, may be had for twelve or fifteen cents a pound. As a rule, however, the camper-out may count on all the trout he cares for without money and without price. Flour, meal, sugar, tea, coffee, canned fruits, and vegetables—all these are sold in the supply store at the hotel, and although the prices range high, the quality of the articles is superior. If the permanency of the camp is definitely fixed upon, it will be well to purchase stores in considerable quantities, thus reducing their cost, as well as the labor of conveying them to camp. In Bloomingdale there is an excellent supply store, where the prices rule considerably lower than in the hotel. To the proprietor of this store, Mr. Isaac Chesley, all orders for provisions may be intrusted, with the certainty of getting what you want, and getting it on reasonable terms.

By no means an unimportant item of expense to those who make any prolonged stay in the woods, is the cost attending the transportation of articles from the outer world. The express charges of the stage lines would seem preposterously high anywhere save in the backwoods. Even here they are much higher than they should be, and, what is worse, they seem to be fixed by no regular schedule, but wholly at the option of the driver. This lack of uniformity leads to no little annoyance. Often we found that the cost of an article was more than doubled by the express charges from Plattsburg to the hotel; and the absurdity of paying forty cents to get a ten-cent tack-hammer brought in from Ausable Forks, reminds one of the purchasing power of Confederate money in 1864. The invalid who depends on friends at home to send him dainties and medicines must be interested in this matter of express charges. Wherever practicable, it is well to use the mail for the transmission of small packages not excluded by the postal rules.

From the foregoing outline of expenses we may formulate some exact estimates as to the cost of camping-out in the Adirondacks. Let us seek first the minimum outlay required to make the experiment.

The patient, we will assume, is poor—so poor that every dime, as well as dollar, must be counted. Suppose him to be a mechanic, with a thrifty, competent, hard-working wife. Suppose him to have been told by a trustworthy physician that his one chance of recovery lies in giving the wilderness cure a trial; that this chance is so large as to amount almost to a certainty, but that if he does not avail himself of it he must inevitably die in a short time. To such a man, living, we will say, in New York or Boston or Philadelphia, Florida would be a mockery, Santa Barbara a dream; but the wilderness invites him, offers him all the benefits which can accrue to anybody, and presents no exorbitant bill for working its marvellous cure. In the estimate that follows, it is assumed that the camp shall consist of a good tent and one bark building; that the invalid's wife shall do the domestic work of the camp, as she has always done of the home; that there shall be an abundance of wholesome food and in greater variety than the poor of our cities can afford; and that, finally, all the essential conditions of the wilderness cure shall be fulfilled as perfectly as if the patient were a rich man. Here are the figures:

Minimum Cost of a Camp for Two Persons, to be Occupied Four Months.

Canvas tent, ...	$25 00
Bark building, ...	10 00
Camp equipments, . . .	15 00
Food and all necessary expenses, per week, $6, . . .	102 00
	$152 00

In the above, no provision is made for the cost of reaching the wilderness nor of the medicines which may be required; neither is there any margin for those delicacies which the invalid is apt to crave; but, nevertheless, the estimate is sufficiently liberal for the making of the experiment under such conditions as have already been explained. Rather than not try the Adirondack cure at all, let the man with $150 and a good wife come along.

Let us pass next to an estimate of the expenses which will be incurred by those persons who are neither rich nor poor—who seek to economize, but are not driven to the stern necessities which pinching poverty demands. Here the comforts of camp life will be considerably increased, and not a few luxuries may be counted upon. The camp itself may include a first class tent and three or four bark buildings; it can employ the steady services of a competent man, who will provide his own boat and attend to all the ordinary labor; it can furnish a table good enough for anybody; and, in short, it can be made home-like and attractive, as an invalid's camp should be. The figures will, I think, in every instance, be found large enough to allow of some little surplus, and the total will be more apt to fall below the estimate than to rise above it. The schedule stands thus:

Medium Cost of a Camp for Two Persons, with Guide, for Four Months.

Canvas tent, ...	$40 00
Building camp, ...	50 00
Equipments, ...	50 00
Food and all necessary expenses, per week, $9, . . .	153 00
Guide for season, . . .	125 00
	$418 00

It should be remembered that in fitting up a camp in the manner supposed in the table above, the health-seeker will have not a little to show at the end of the season in the line of equipments. If he decides to remain through a second or third summer, comparatively little money will need to be added to the original outlay. On the other hand, if he is able to go out of the woods at the end of his first season, he can easily dispose of all his camp adjuncts at a fair price.

Although anything like a precise calculation of the amount of money which *might* be spent in this wilderness experiment would be as impossible to make

as it would to determine the sum Sinbad might
have spent in those years which intervened between
his rash demand for the roc's egg and his happy
death, nevertheless, an approximation to the possible
extravagance of life in the woods may properly be
added.   And here it is:

*Maximum Cost of a Camp for Two Persons, and
Guides, for Four Months.*

Canvas tents, ...	$100 00
Building camp, . . .	250 00
Equipments, ...	250 00
Wages, five men and one woman (all "guides"), . . .	1,200 00
Running expenses, . . .	500 00
	$2,300 00

Here, of course, the "maximum" is that of the
probable, not by any means of the possible.   The
Count of Monte Christo might fashion his tent of
camel's-hair, and floor his bark cabins with the cedar
of Lebanon.   He might spend as much money in the
woods as in Paris; but he would not recover his
health any the quicker for that.   The maximum estimate presumes extravagance, but it does not exceed
the actual outlay which has been made by campers-
out in the Adirondacks.

So much for the cost of one part of the wilderness
experiment.   For the other—the winter residence—
it may easily be shown that the cost of living is con-

siderably less than at the long-established health resorts; while to the person willing to economize, it is
a simple matter to materially reduce the amount
usually expended by health-seekers.

In Saranac Lake, superior accommodation may
be had for $20 a week for two persons. The smaller
houses fix their prices at from $14 to $16 per week
for two. In Bloomingdale, fair board can be obtained anywhere from $12 to $20 per week, while in
the farm-houses scattered over the country, the winter sojourner may find a home for the price—little
or much—he is able to pay. His own experience in
this matter was so pleasant, that it may naturally
prejudice the writer in favor of farm-house board;
but others, less fortunate in the selection of a place,
might find it wearisome.

But the winter may be passed in the woods at a
much smaller outlay than boarding in any way ne-
cessitates. Let us take up our mechanic again, who,
with the coming of the keen November days, finds
the promise of recovery already half-fulfilled. Whatever sacrifice a continued stay may call for, he must
not think of leaving the woods now. All his progress will come to naught if he refuses to give nature
time to work out her miracles in her own way. Six
or seven months longer and he may go back with a
twenty years' lease of life. It is worth some pinching to get a grip on a lease of that sort. So the man
who is absolutely poor puts the thoughts of board
out of his mind, rents a small house a mile perhaps
from his camp, furnishes it with the equipments of

7

the latter, and such additional articles as he can make
with his own hands, and is prepared to brave the
winter in comfort and independence. A house with
enough room to decently accommodate two, or even
four persons, can be rented for $2 a month. It is a
backwoods house to be sure, most likely of logs, but
still inhabitable—a palace to the tenement prisons of
New York. It is lacking all modern nuisances. The
atmosphere within it may be kept almost as pure and
fresh as that outside. An abundance of wood for
fuel to keep two stoves roaring through the cold season can be bought for $10, or for something less than
a dollar a cord. Here, then, are the two important
items of shelter and fuel provided for at a total outlay of $24 for the full seven months. In the matter
of food, a plain, nourishing, abundant diet can be
furnished for two persons at an expense of $4 a week.
This would allow of good bread and butter, mutton,
beef, sausages, ham, fish, potatoes, beans, peas, turnips, cabbages, milk, all in generous quantities, and
with now and then some dainty from the outer-world
market. Allow twenty-five cents a week for light,
another twenty-five for a good daily newspaper, and
fifty for the heathen—or tobacco. This gives us a
total, with the house-rent and fuel, of something over
$6 a week for all ordinary household expenditures!

Where, the country over, can the mechanic and
his wife live for less than that?

If it shall seem to the general reader that this
matter of cost has been entered into with too great
minuteness of detail, let it charitably be remembered

that in a large number of cases it is the question which must determine the invalid's course. We should not all be rich, even if the bricks which pave Boston were turned suddenly to gold. There would be plenty of bricks, but we could not all get to Boston. So when Hope points the way to the weary victim of wasting disease, but points always and only to those distant heights he can never mount, what a solace is it to know that others more lucky have found the treasure he coveted, but could not seek? Here, in the vast wilderness, that treasure may be searched for anew. And this little book will have fulfilled its modest mission if it carries aught of aid, or cheer, or comfort to the sick.

APPENDIX.

Although nearly everything necessary for the building and equipping of a camp has been mentioned in the preceding pages, it may, nevertheless, be a convenience to the reader if the essential articles are grouped together under a single heading. First, then, for the

Necessities.

1 cook-stove.

1 tent-stove, with at least four lengths of pipe.

1 tea-kettle.

1 iron pot, for boiling.

1 broiler, for meat.

1 baking-pan.

1 frying-pan.

1 coffee-pot.

Heavy stone-ware crockery, number of pieces to be determined by number of persons.

6 tin pails, from two to sixteen quarts in size.

Knives and forks, spoons, and carving-knife and fork.

6 tin cups.
6 tin bread-pans of different sizes.
2 market-baskets.
4 candlesticks.
1 lantern.
1 hatchet.
1 axe.
1 hammer.
1 hand-saw.

With regard to the provisions and stores, the
amount to be expended will, as has already been intimated, depend largely upon the taste and means of
the camper-out. The subjoined tables may serve to
convey an approximate idea of what will be needed.

A Minimum Estimate.

Flour, 1 bag.
Sugar, 20 pounds.
Yeast, or yeast cakes.
Baking-powder.
Salt, pepper, etc.
Potatoes.
Salt pork.
Tea and coffee.
Indian-meal.
Beans.
Candles—kerosene, or both.
Matches—a goodly supply.
Crackers.

To the above list, if one cares to give himself a little larger variety of food and some additional comforts, may be added the following, which we will call

A Moderate Estimate.

All that is contained under the minimum estimate.
1 dozen canned tomatoes.
1 dozen canned corn.
1 dozen canned fruit to suit the taste.
Ham.
1 dozen chickens (to be bought alive and kept in camp).
½ dozen boxes sardines.
Pressed corn-beef.
Cheese.
Dried beef.
Lager-beer.*

To those who may desire a still more varied menu, here is a list which may be helpful in making out the schedule of stores.

A Luxurious Estimate.

All that is contained under the preceding heads.
Canned lobster, salmon, shrimps, etc.
Clam-chowder, pickled oysters, chow-chow, etc.

---

* So many consumptive patients take lager-beer regularly, under advice of their physicians, that it is regarded almost a necessity in their diet. The writer found it a great saving to buy his lager by the keg in Plattsburg and bottle it in camp. It kept excellently buried in the sand. Empty bottles can be had at the hotel.

Canned soups, turtle, chicken, beef, etc.
Potted meats.
Canned fruits and vegetables to suit taste.
Olives, pickles and relishes to taste.
Wine.

With regard to milk, butter, and eggs, these, as has been heretofore suggested, may best be procured of the nearest farmer.

As to the quantity of provisions to be taken into camp, the invalid must, of course, use his own discretion. If there be but two in the party with the guide, enough of the staple articles to last a fortnight will do to begin with. After a little experience it may be advantageous to buy on a larger scale.

I have already sought to point out what is and what is not necessary in the way of wearing apparel. All advice on this may be epitomized in a single sentence :—Take as little as you can consistent with comfort, and let that little be all available. Plenty of woollen and flannel, either for man or woman, is the golden rule.

The reader has fully discovered that this little volume is not a sportsman's book ; but as many a patient may be strong enough to amuse himself with gun and rod, I append the following

SPORTING OUTFIT.

One rifle (a shotgun is of no use, except for partridge-hunting, and a rifle answers equally well even for that).

Ammunition, a moderate supply. You can refill your cartridge-box any time at the hotel.

One fly-rod. If you choose you can buy it in the wilderness; or, if you are a beginner, you may save some considerable loss by learning to cast a fly with a tamarack pole, which can be cut anywhere.

One landing-net.

An assortment of flies.

With regard to these last, I cannot do better than quote the advice of the Rev. Mr. Murray, who ought to be an authority on trout-fishing. He says: "Take of hackles six each, of black, red, and brown. Let the flies be made on hooks from Nos. 3 to 1, Limerick size. In addition to the hackles, take six Canada flies, six green drakes, six red ibis, six small salmon flies, and, if in the fall of the year, six English bluejay and six gray drake."

The cost of the above fishing outfit ought not to exceed $25.

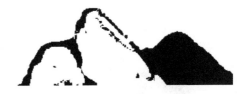

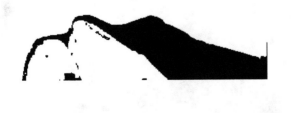